Dedication

To Julia and Ffion:

'Pooh,' he whispered. 'Yes Piglet?' 'Nothing,' said Piglet, taking Pooh's paw, 'I just wanted to be sure of you.'

A. A. Milne, *The House at Pooh Corner*

When the News is Bad

A GUIDE FOR HEALTH PROFESSIONALS ON BREAKING BAD NEWS

Ann Faulkner
Communication in Health Care, The Mount,
Causeway Head Road, Sheffield S17 3DY

Stanley Thornes (Publishers) Ltd

First published in 1998 by:
Stanley Thornes (Publishers) Ltd
Ellenborough House
Wellington Street
CHELTENHAM
GL50 1YW
United Kingdom

98 99 00 01 / 10 9 8 7 6 5 4 3 2 1

A catalogue record for this book is available from the British Library

ISBN 0-7487-3345-0

Typeset by Acorn Bookwork, Salisbury, Wiltshire
Printed and bound in Great Britain
by T.J. International Ltd, Padstow, Cornwall

Contents

Preface

In the early years of my concerns for patient care, the answer appeared to lie in improving communication between patients, relatives, and those who cared for them. It has been both exhilarating and rewarding to be involved in an area where change has gathered pace to the extent that there is now a universal push to put communication in all medical and nursing curricula.

This increased recognition has brought a further refinement in that specific areas of need are being identified. One of these is the problem of handling bad news situations. Here, there is an increasing demand from doctors, nurses, and other health professionals for help in improving the way that bad news is given. This book responds to that need and has been written to provide a practical guide for those in health care who wish to improve their skills and develop strategies to handle bad news situations and to deal with the aftermath.

Throughout the book are exercises which aim to develop reflective practice, enhance insight, and improve self awareness. They can be used by an individual working alone, or by a tutor to encourage discussion and where participants in training may choose to share their thoughts and feelings. As in all situations with the potential for bad news, there are no magic answers; what I hope I have achieved is a book that will allow the individual to deal with bad news situations in a sensitive and useful way.

Ann Faulkner, 1997

Acknowledgements

My beliefs about breaking bad news originated from my clinical work and were later reinforced by the joint work undertaken with Peter Maguire. This book reflects the lessons learned from that period and the subsequent work with colleagues at Trent Palliative Care Centre. My particular thanks to Catherine O'Keeffe, Avril Jones, and Jackie Argent for their support, to my family, and especially to Barbara Grimbley for her patience in typing the manuscript.

Introduction

There has been increasing concern in recent years about the way in which bad news is broken in healthcare. Patients particularly seem to remember bad news situations in detail, even some considerable time after the event (Hogbin, Jenkins and Parkin, 1992; Faulkner, Peace and O'Keefe, 1995a). Health professionals appear to be similarly concerned about how bad news should be broken (Gray, 1992; Fallowfield, 1993).

It is very common to predict, often without relevant information, how a person might react in a given situation. Bad news is an example of this, with assumptions being made about what *is* bad news and the effect that it is likely to have on the recipient. It is often assumed, for example, that when one partner in a relationship dies, this is going to be the worst news possible for the survivor. In fact, the couple may have been living together for many years for a variety of reasons that do not include love. It may be that they were responsible for their children and the awareness that those children needed two parents kept them together even though they no longer liked each other. It could also be, particularly for a woman who did not work, that she stayed in a relationship because she could not afford to get out of it. In those situations the death of the partner, particularly if it brings financial security and independence, may not be bad news at all.

Alternatively it may be assumed that death will be a relief rather than bad news, when one partner has cared for the other throughout a long and difficult illness. In fact the death may devastate the surviving partner since caring for the beloved had become their *raison d'être* and the death may have created an enormous gap.

We may also assume that a severe and potentially life-threatening diagnosis will constitute bad news for the recipient. Again, this may not be the case. The patient who has been feeling poorly and unwell for a long time without a diagnosis, or feeling that she has not been understood by her doctor, may have an overwhelming sense of relief when a diagnosis is made. In such a case one might expect that a later reaction could be dismay at the uncertainty of the future but the initial response may be 'Thank goodness that I have got something the matter with me – I was beginning to think I was neurotic.'

For other individuals a life-threatening illness can bring secondary gains. The patient who is lonely and feels that nobody cares much about them may find that illness brings attention from people who were otherwise rather cool. This was certainly the case for Eva who, after her diagnosis of cancer, found that her overcritical mother became far more caring and that her disinterested colleagues at work began to pay her attention.

Given the above and the vast differences between individuals and what is and is not important to them, how is it possible to define 'bad news'? One definition may be that bad news is information that could radically change the life of the recipient. In fact, this could equally apply to good news, such as winning the lottery, where the impact of the news may be so overwhelming that the individual finds it very difficult to absorb at the point of delivery. That both bad and good news can change an individual's life requires that the definition of bad news has an extra dimension. It is suggested here that bad news is any information that the recipient does not wish to hear. Such a definition means that with some messages it will not be possible to tell at the point of delivery whether they constitute good or bad news. This theme will be further developed in Chapter 2. What is important is that no judgement should be made about a situation until facts are known, not only about the patient or recipient of the news, but also about events surrounding the situation. A theme throughout this book will be the need to assess the recipient's reactions to information about diagnosis, prognosis or treatment options.

WHY IS BREAKING BAD NEWS DIFFICULT?

There is a general consensus that breaking bad news is difficult and something that most health professionals do not wish to do. Part of this may be because giving someone a diagnosis of a condition that may be life-threatening and for which there may be no cure, goes against the ideals of good practice. As one sixth-year medical student described it, 'From the day you start being a medical student, you're taught that the essence of being a good doctor is to make a rapid and accurate diagnosis, prescribe appropriate treatment and send the patient home well. Against a background like that it's very difficult to tell somebody that they won't get well. After all, what good news message can you possibly give them?'

Certainly doctors do not appear to be taught how to break bad news. Faulkner and colleagues (1995b) found that doctors were unsure where to break the bad news, how to break it, and how to deal with the collusion that often followed the breaking of bad news to relatives rather than the patient. The doctors also expressed their feelings of helplessness when they could not follow bad news with any positive offers for the future. Another feature of this study was that the doctors concerned appeared to take responsibility for the bad news. This links with the ancient Greeks' philosophy which was to shoot the bearer of bad tidings and in some way make him the responsible person for the message that he brought. There are many areas in medicine where patients are given bad news and uncertainty because of the state of the art of medicine and the need for further scientific development. This knowledge should help doctors to realize that medicine does not yet have all the answers, but it seems not to take away from the awful sense of responsibility when telling an individual that their life expectancy is much less than was previously thought, or that they may never recover total good health.

Given the above, it could be argued that in sudden death situations such as road traffic accidents that there is less of a sense of responsibility. Even so, the fact that the young man who had a motorcycle accident cannot be revived is again taken on the shoulders of the health professional, given the belief that the doctor's role is to cure.

Perhaps the greatest difficulty in breaking bad news is having to face someone and tell them something that they may find extremely painful. The overwhelming feeling of helplessness makes breaking bad news very difficult indeed.

WHOSE RESPONSIBILITY?

'Who should break bad news?' is a common question from health professionals at all levels. It could be argued that in the case of diagnosis then the bearer of the bad tidings should be the consultant. Junior doctors, however, often complain that the consultant passes the buck so that they are left to break bad news to patients they do not know, and often without the necessary information to handle the difficult questions which may follow when bad news has been broken.

When the bad news is of a death, then it may be broken by a variety of personnel including the police for accidental death, and any member of the healthcare team for death in a hospital or hospice.

In fact the responsibility for breaking bad news should rest with a member of staff with whom the recipient can feel comfortable. This means that any member of the healthcare team should be prepared to give information at a time the patient is ready for it even if that information is life threatening. Such a belief has implications for the training of all members of the caring professions.

TO TELL OR NOT TO TELL

Many years ago there was considerable debate on whether an individual should be told or not told a life-threatening diagnosis and poor prognosis. The group who felt that the patient should not be told took the paternalistic view that patients and their relatives may not be strong enough to receive bad news. Those who felt that patients should be told tended to talk about the individual needing to face reality. That debate no longer seems to be a large issue. It is accepted that the individual has a right to information about his disease and its treatment. In spite of that there are still patients who argue that they are not told their diagnosis and that they do not understand their treatment.

It would be easy to argue that the patient who does not understand his disease and its treatment has not been told in an effective way. In fact, what may be more important is not what has or has not been said but what the patient has understood. There are many cancer patients who are relieved to be told that they have 'a little tumour'. By using euphemisms like this the patient is allowed to reject the word 'cancer' and convince themselves that that is not their diagnosis. It is argued here that if bad news is broken effectively, then the recipient will absorb the major items of that message *if he is ready to do so*.

Another issue in whether or not to tell an individual bad news is the fact that many people may not wish to hear the news or be ready to absorb it. In the case of a sudden death there is little choice. The reality has to be faced. But in life-threatening illness and an uncertain prognosis then one could argue that the individual has the right to reject or delay hearing the information. This will be explored in Chapter 6.

WHO TO TELL?

One could argue that there is no question who should receive bad news. It should be the individual who is most affected by that news. In healthcare this may be the patient. In sudden death situations it is the next of kin, i.e. the partner or nearest blood relative. Both of these above assumptions can cause problems.

The patient

Information about diagnosis and prognosis legally belongs to the patient. However, medical staff do have the right to decide that a patient may not be able to deal with the situation and may then choose to tell a relative first. Another reason for telling the relative is that many doctors find it less painful to give the news 'once removed'. Junior doctors at lunchtime seminars admit that it is easier to tell the relative than to face the patient with a life-threatening disease.

It can be argued that the doctor should not tell the relative first and that the patient should be aware of their rights. Doctors could be seen to be taking a professional risk if they disclose information to another that actually belongs to the patient. In fact reality often makes things difficult for a doctor. Relatives may be very demanding and ask a lot of questions. This can put the doctor into a very difficult situation, for if he refuses to talk it could be seen that he may be covering something up. On the other hand, if he gives the information to the relative the patient may well be very upset.

A further difficulty may arise if the patient is frankly uninterested in their diagnosis and the doctor feels that somebody in the family must know what the current situation is.

It can be seen that giving information can be fraught with difficulties unless something is known of the patient and his or her relationships and needs for accurate information.

Relatives

When a patient is married or has a partner, it is assumed that the next of kin is that partner and if the patient is unable to absorb bad news, the partner is seen to be the most appropriate person to be informed. If the patient does not have a partner then the appropriate person is seen to be either a parent or a sibling.

In fact, if possible it is vital to find out from the patient who the most appropriate person is to have information. Those working with AIDS will know that often the most appropriate person for information is the homosexual partner, who may not be recognized by the immediate family of the patient. In order that information is given to the appropriate person it is necessary to know who that person actually is. Even when such information is available there may be difficulties within and between families over who is the person most responsible.

SUMMARY

In this introduction, the general issues around breaking bad news have been considered. The need for a definition of bad news has been addressed, as has the problem of why it is so difficult to tell people things that they do not want to hear. It has been suggested that, although in certain instances there is one person responsible for breaking bad news, all those in the caring professions may be faced with this responsibility and therefore need to develop relevant skills. Finally, the decision to tell or not to tell has been considered, along with the difficulty of making the right decision about who to tell.

EXERCISE

A patient is expecting to be discharged from hospital, but the consultant decides that further investigations are necessary. He has not yet spoken to her. The patient asks you if she will be able to go home this week.

- *How do you react?*
- *What would you say?*
- *How do you think you would feel in this situation?*

REFERENCES

Fallowfield, L. (1993) Giving bad and sad news, *Lancet*, **341**, 476–8.

Faulkner, A., Peace, G. and O'Keeffe, C. (1995a) *Child of a Dying Parent*, Chapman and Hall, London.

Faulkner A., Argent, J., Jones, A. and O'Keeffe, C. (1995b) Improving the skills of doctors in giving distressing information. *Medical Information*, **29**(4), 303–7.

Gray. M. A. (1992) Cancer, the dreaded diagnosis. *Care of the Critically Ill*, **8**(4), 161–3.

Hogbin, B., Jenkins, V. A. and Parkin, A. (1992) Remembering 'bad news' consultations. *Psycho-Oncology*, **1**, 147–54.

Breaking bad news | 2

Except for unexpected trauma, such as death and disaster, few individuals will be entirely unprepared for bad news. For example, the individual who goes to his general practitioner usually has symptoms that are giving him concern. He may have difficulty in passing urine or be getting pains that have not been present before. Given his symptoms it is highly unlikely that the patient will present at the general practitioner's in a totally neutral frame of mind. Consider the case of Mr Timms:

> Mr Timms found blood when he went to the toilet. He had been a little constipated so felt that the bleeding was probably because he had had to strain to pass his stool. Later he noticed that he passed blood even when he was not constipated. His cousin, Dick, had symptoms the year before and had been diagnosed with bowel cancer so when Mr Timms went to his general practitioner, the fear in the back of his mind was that he in fact was suffering from bowel cancer and might need a colostomy.

Such fears are not always verbalized unless the doctor makes a real assessment of why the patient has come to him on this particular day. The doctor may assume that the patient has no idea of the significance of the blood that he is passing, in which case he will lose the opportunity to identify where the patient is coming from in terms of his fears and worries. By assessing the patient's concern the doctor is then able to put his own potential diagnosis into context for the patient (Faulkner, 1997). This may mean an opportunity to reassure the patient that the matter may not be as serious as he fears or to warn him that the possibility that he is considering is a very real one. For example:

Doctor: Well Mr Timms, what can I do for you today?

Mr Timms: Well doc, I'm a bit worried. I've been passing blood when I go to the toilet.

Doctor: Can you tell me some more about that?

Mr Timms: Well, I thought first of all it was because I was constipated but I had diarrhoea last week and still was passing blood.

Doctor: And what's your main concern, Mr Timms?

Mr Timms: Well, my cousin was like this and his was cancer.

Doctor: Well, I'm sorry to tell you this but that's one possibility, but only one. There are many more simple things that can be causing your bleeding so I think what we're going to have to do is to get some investigations done.

In the above exchange, the patient has felt that he is heard and that his concerns are realistic. At the same time, he has had a certain measure of reassurance that there could be other reasons why he is passing blood. Of course some patients may have no idea of the problem that underlies their symptoms. The symptoms may be totally outside their experience, either personally or within their family and friendship circle. When a patient with no information or beliefs about their illness sees the doctor, it is still worth asking that patient what they feel is happening.

Doctor: Well Miss Avery, what can I do for you today?

Miss Avery: I'm not sure doctor but I'm very, very worried.

Doctor: Well, tell me something about your worry.

Miss Avery: Well, it's nothing I can put my finger on. I'm just tired all the time and although I wanted to lose some weight, I've tried oh so many times, so many diets, and now suddenly without any effort I'm losing weight.

Doctor: And how does all this seem to you?

Miss Avery: Well that's why I'm here, I just don't understand what it's all about and, you know, I'm worried to death that I might just be neurotic and I just don't know how to pull myself together.

In the above exchange the patient had two major symptoms – one of tiredness and one of loss of weight – and yet within her own experience she could not relate any potential diagnosis to her symptoms except that she might be somehow responsible for her lethargy and negative feelings. As with Mr Timms, the doctor may have ideas of what is causing the symptoms but will wish to get the patient examined by a specialist before any decisions are made.

THE WARNING SHOT

When an individual is entirely unprepared for bad news, either because that news is totally unexpected or because the individual has not been able to make sense of the symptoms that they have, it helps to give some warning that the news may be bad.

The doctor or nurse may give a non-verbal warning that

they have serious news by looking grave and concerned. However, this in itself could be misinterpreted by an anxious patient or, indeed, not noticed. Doctors and nurses, on the whole, are accepted by society as people who will make bad things better. The police, on the other hand, are associated with keeping law and order and are only seen personally by members of the public in a bad news situation. Opening the front door to a policeman dressed in his uniform is a powerful warning shot that something serious is about to be discussed. Doctors, nurses, and other health professionals do not have such a strong non-verbal cue and must learn to use appropriate words that will alert the recipient to the forthcoming news without frightening them so that they are in a state of high anxiety. For example, the doctor, when talking to Mr Timms, did not deny that his fears could be well-founded but what the doctor did do was point out that without investigations, several other diagnoses were possible. The doctor did not gloss over Mr Timm's concerns but when the point of diagnosis arrives, he will be sure that Mr Timms has had some warning that his worst fears may prove to be true.

In spite of Mr Timms' knowledge that cancer of the bowel is a possible diagnosis, when the results of his investigations come out, whoever gives him the news will again need to re-warn him if, indeed, the diagnosis is bowel cancer.

Doctor: Good morning Mr Timms.

Mr Timms: Good morning. I'm very worried about these
            investigations you did because I'm still
            passing blood.

Doctor: I've got these results for you now and I have
            to warn you that the news is serious.

Mr Timms: So it's cancer then?

Doctor: I'm afraid so.

Because Mr Timms had had a warning, both from his general practitioner and from his consultant, he was able to leap immediately from the warning shot to the actual news. This often happens particularly when the patient has their own theories about what is wrong with them.

Miss Avery, on the other hand, who did not know what her diagnosis was would need much more help through the process of learning that her condition was relatively serious.

FINDING THE RIGHT WORDS

There are no right words for breaking bad news. However, there are a number of general principles that allow bad news to be broken in a sensitive way that the recipient can understand (Maguire, Faulkner and Regnard, 1995). By assessing the situation and giving a warning shot, one may prepare a patient for information that they may find very distressing. An important principle is to keep the news as succinct and clear as possible. There is a danger of giving too much information and putting the patient or relative into a state of information overload where almost nothing will be remembered (Centeno-Cortes and Nunez-Olarte, 1994). Compare the following exchanges:

(1)

Doctor: Well Miss Avery, we have the results of our investigations and I'm afraid they are more serious than we hoped.

Miss Avery: More serious?

Doctor: Yes, I'm afraid that you've got a type of anaemia.

Miss Avery: Well that's alright, isn't it? It's iron pills for anaemia.

Doctor:	Well this particular sort of anaemia will need more than iron tablets.
Miss Avery:	But you can make me better?
Doctor:	We can certainly improve your health dramatically with appropriate treatment. Do you want me to explain the situation?

(2)

Doctor:	Miss Avery, I have the results of your tests. I'm afraid it's pretty serious.
Miss Avery:	Serious?
Doctor:	Yes, I'm afraid you've got anaemia of a chronic sort.
Miss Avery:	But I thought with anaemia you just cure it with iron tablets. Perhaps I've been eating the wrong diet.
Doctor:	No, you have what we call pernicious anaemia and that comes as a result of Vitamin B12 deficiency. There are many causes for this...

In the first scenario the doctor was concerned to work at the patient's pace in giving information. This means that on the day the news is broken the patient may absorb only the knowledge that things are serious. However, the patient will have the opportunity to go back or to talk to a nurse and gradually fill in the missing information. If one works at the patient's pace in this way, the news is much more likely to be absorbed.

In the second exchange the doctor went straight into a description of the chronic disease. In the shock of hearing that the news is serious, the patient is unlikely to remember more than a fraction of what the doctor said.

In both scenarios the patient is likely to leave the doctor with the remembrance that the problem is due to anaemia. In the first scenario the door is open for the patient to go back and ask questions and get information at their own pace. In the second scenario the doctor will feel that he has given the patient all the information that she needs and this will make it more difficult for the patient to feel able to ask more questions at a later date.

In many bad news situations it is not necessary for the individual to have any more information than they feel able to handle at one time (Greger, 1993). Sudden death or disaster constrains the model, for although there are many parallels there is not the luxury of allowing the recipient to choose the amount of information, or the time scale, in the same way. Doctors may argue that in busy clinics and outpatients departments, or even on the wards, there is not the time to work at the patient's pace. But if news is given in manageable chunks it can be given over time and it may be that the person who gives the basic news – e.g. to Mrs Avery that she has anaemia – may not be the person who later answers her questions about her own particular type of anaemia and what that will mean to her life and the way she lives it. The alternative is a patient who has been given all the information they need but in a way that will not stay with them and could lead to problems later as they misinterpret their treatment regimen.

CUES

Just as doctors give non-verbal signals along with their verbal messages, so do the patients. In breaking bad news, it is important to observe the patients' reactions and the cues they give us about what those reactions are or, before that, what they expect the news to be. The patient may look anxious or very worried, or may appear to be very nervous. In order to interpret these cues properly, it is necessary to acknowledge that they are there. Making an educated guess gives the patient the opportunity to confirm that, yes, that is how they feel, or, no, that is not how they feel, and in the latter instance to elaborate how they do actually feel. For example:

Doctor: You are looking very worried, Mr Timms.

Mr Timms: Well, not exactly worried, more thinking ahead and it just doesn't look too good.

Doctor: What do you mean by that?

Mr Timms: Well, like I told you, Dick was dead in three months.

Here, by acknowledging the non-verbal cues from Mr Timms, the doctor gained more information about the way that the patient was interpreting his diagnosis of cancer of the bowel, and this allowed him to give realistic reassurance on the expected outcomes in Mr Timms' case.

There may be fear on the part of the health professional to acknowledge non-verbal behaviour because the interpretation may be incorrect. In fact most patients are very appreciative of the fact that the health professional is taking an interest in them and are well able to affirm or correct the assumption that is being tested out by the health professional.

In deciding on the level of information to give, the patient's cues can help the health professional considerably. Miss Avery, for example, gave the cue that she knew something about anaemia in that she felt it could be cured by taking iron tablets. However, had she known more than that simple fact it could well have come out in verbal cues, as follows:

Doctor: Yes, I'm afraid that you've got a type of anaemia.

Miss Avery: Anaemia – what sort of anaemia?

By asking this question, Miss Avery gives a very strong cue that she knows that there is more than one type of anaemia and, further, that she is ready to hear about her own. Similarly, the patient can give cues that the doctor is going too fast:

Mr Timms: So it's cancer then?

Doctor: I'm afraid so. Can I give you some indication of what we can do in your particular case?

Mr Timms: Well, all I really want to know is whether you can cure it.

In the above exchange, Mr Timms made it clear that his need for information was concerned with possible treatment and cure. This allowed the doctor to continue to work at Mr Timms' pace. By tailoring news in this way, one enables patients to absorb appropriate information at a pace that is comfortable for them. This may mean that many patients leave the doctor with only minimal knowledge of what is wrong, but if the situation is followed up and information given when the patient is ready for it the bad news is more likely to be absorbed and the patient more likely to adapt to the altered situation in his life.

Even when bad news is expected, there is the possibility of shock. It is almost as if the hope that things will be all right is maintained until the very last minute. Mr Timms, for example, hoped that, although his symptoms suggested cancer as a possibility, that this would not be so. He had spent many hours, in the few days between the investigations and his next appointment with the doctor, imagining all sorts of things that could happen but was always able to shake himself out of it by feeling that he was being overpessimistic. Even though he was able to say, 'So it's cancer', to the doctor, when it was confirmed that he did indeed have bowel cancer, Mr Timms was in a state of shock. In being aware of this the doctor could avoid giving too much information and so give the necessary space for the news to be properly absorbed.

WORKING TO A STRUCTURE

Following a structure for breaking bad news has two positive effects. Firstly, it allows the health professional to break bad news without doing psychological damage to the patient and, secondly, it leaves the patient in control of the rate at which they receive the news. Figure 2.1 shows a diagram of the structure suggested in this book. The health professional using such a structure will need the skills to allow the patient to set the pace and to verbalize their reactions. It can be criticized because it also allows the patient to stop the interaction at any time when they feel they do not wish for more information. This can lead to denial, which will be considered in Chapter 6.

By leaving the patient in control of the pace at which he learns the news, the structure can be very compressed or very elongated. In fact some patients may not ever know the true nature of their disease and one can argue that this is their right. What is important is that the patient can express clearly how they feel so that the health professional does not push more information towards the patient than they can manage at a particular time.

Figure 2.1   Strategy for breaking bad news

Strategy	Example	
(1) Identify current knowledge or suspicions.	Doctor:	What sense are you making of this?
(a) None	(a) Patient:	That's what's so worrying – none of it makes sense.
(b) Some	(b) Patient:	Well, my mum had something similar and hers was arthritis.
(2) Warn of impending news (warning shot).	(a) Doctor:	I can see how worried you are. I can't say much until we have run some tests, but you are right to take this seriously.
	(b) Doctor:	I'm afraid you could be right, but let's get some investigations done and then we can look at options.
(3) News at patient's pace and in manageable chunks.	Doctor:	We have the results of your tests and I'm afraid it *is* serious.
	Patient:	How serious?
(4) Allow patient to choose when they have heard enough.	Patient:	So, it's my waterworks?
	Doctor:	Yes, I'd like to explain the situation.
	Patient:	No thanks – just tell me what you can do about it. I doubt I'd understand the mechanics.
(5) Give space.		
(6) Handle reactions.	Doctor:	This must have been difficult for you – can you tell me how you are feeling?

Source: Faulkner, 1997.

Conversely, there are patients who collapse the structure by demanding information in a direct and straightforward way:

Miss Potts: It's diabetes, isn't it doctor – all this running to the toilet and feeling so dry and losing weight?

Doctor: It certainly sounds like it but let's wait until the nurse comes back with the results of testing your urine.

Miss Potts: How would you treat it? Is it going to be injections for the rest of my life. Oh God, I hope not.

The above case could be as difficult to handle as the case of the patient who has no knowledge of the news that is about to be broken. Miss Potts was a dietician with considerable knowledge. She had worked out for herself what her diagnosis was likely to be and had come to the doctor armed with that knowledge. However, there is still the possibility that when the nurse comes back with the results of the urine test that Miss Potts could get very distressed. The doctor delayed agreeing to the potential diagnosis until he had the evidence in front of him. This also acted as a pause for Miss Potts to get more worries out of her system before the nurse came back. Even with patients who have worked out the probable diagnosis and prognosis, there still remains a small hope that their fears are unfounded, and so the experience of shock remains a possibility for the health professional to handle.

THE NEED FOR SPACE

Given that even expected unpleasant news can result in some level of shock, the major requirement of most individuals when bad news has been broken is for some space where they can try to absorb what has been said and make some sense of it in the context of their own lives. There appears to be an overwhelming need on the part of health professionals to follow bad news with some sort of positive message. For this reason, they tend not to give space after bad news is broken but to move into giving information, preferably of a positive type. Work with members of the police force (Faulkner, Argent and Craig, 1994) showed that although they had problems in breaking bad news at the patient's pace, they seemed to have a clear understanding of the need for space after the news had been given. Making the recipient a cup of tea was considered almost a duty by the police. This has two functions: one, it leaves the individual on their own for a short time while the drink is being made, but, secondly, it also seems to bring some level of comfort as they struggle to absorb what has been said to them. What seems common to all bad news situations is that information given immediately after bad news is broken is unlikely to be remembered.

The constraints of time are often given as a reason why it is not possible to give space to an individual after bad news has been broken. Of increasing concern in outpatients departments are the facilities that are available for people who have to wait when their relative has been brought in after an accident (Faulkner and Lilley, 1996). Bad news is often given bluntly and the relative left to handle their reactions without appropriate support.

SUMMARY

In this chapter the structure of breaking bad news has been addressed along with consideration of the words to use when telling an individual something that they do not wish to hear. The concept of assessment and of giving a warning shot have also been explored along with the necessity of working at the recipient's pace. The notion of shock has been explored in terms of the effect on the individual of a message that constitutes bad news.

EXERCISE

A patient is diagnosed with a potentially serious disease, but is not asking questions or appearing to be interested in her diagnosis. How would you:

- *Assess the patient's current belief or knowledge about her illness?*
- *Decide on how much information to give to the patient?*

REFERENCES

Centeno-Cortes, C. and Nunez-Olarte, J. M. (1994) Questioning diagnosis disclosure in terminal cancer patients. *Palliative Medicine*, 8(1), 39–44.

Faulkner, A. (1997) *Effective Interaction with Patients*, 2nd edn, Churchill Livingstone, Edinburgh.

Faulkner, A., Argent, J. and Craig, B. (1994) Interacting effectively with the public: the effect of skill based workshops on police constables. Occasional Paper No. 12, Trent Palliative Care Centre, Sheffield.

Faulkner, A. and Lilley, R. (1996) *Bereavement: A Management Check List*. Published privately. Available from: Communication in Health Care, The Mount, Sheffield S17 3DY.

Greger, H. A. (1993) When is ignorance bliss? The effects of knowledge on quality of life among socio-economically disadvantaged cancer patients. *Diss. Abstr. Int. A.*, 54(1), 321.

Maguire, P., Faulkner, A. and Regnard, C. (1995) Breaking bad news: a flow diagram, in *Flow Diagrams in Advanced Cancer and Other Diseases* (eds C. Regnard and J. Hockley), Edward Arnold, London.

Picking up the pieces 3

It was seen in Chapter 2 that even when an individual is prepared for bad news, such as the impending death of a relative, a sense of shock and unreality is still likely to be present when the news is actually spelt out. This will happen no matter how well or badly the news has been broken. It does seem that one of the attributes of human nature is to hold on to hope, even in a hopeless situation, until the very last minute. This is why relatives often seem quite stunned by the news that a loved person has died after a long illness when the death was expected. It is only after such news has been absorbed that any effort can be made to pick up the pieces and help the individual to adapt to the inevitable change that the news will bring.

Health professionals do not appear to be comfortable with silence after a bad news message. Faulkner and colleagues (1995) found that doctors who were breaking bad news in a simulated situation were at great pains to give patients a positive message following bad news about a diagnosis and prognosis. Only 5% of the doctors in this study actually gave the patient any mental space. The majority of doctors went immediately into giving information about treatment options and the future. Many of these doctors gave overoptimistic reassurance rather than a realistic message.

Some would argue that such optimism is necessary in order to give the patient a positive message to take away (Brewin, 1996), but this view does not sit well with current research findings that the majority of patients prefer a realistic message (Williams, 1996).

If possible, a quiet place should be found for the patients to sit while they come to grips with what has happened. Some outpatients departments provide voluntary sitters for those who are waiting for news of someone who has been brought in critically ill or for those whose relative has been brought in dead on arrival. The function of these sitters is not to talk but to be there for the individual while they absorb the bad news.

In a busy hospital it is often difficult to find a space where someone can have the privacy to cry if necessary, or just to sit and let the news sink in. However, it usually is possible to create the illusion of privacy or to find a quiet corner where the individual can sit. Later there will be all sorts of questions that need to be asked but in the initial period of shock the likelihood is that just the one most important word is going round and round in the individual's mind. It may be 'cancer' as a diagnosis, it might be 'death' after a road traffic accident, but for the moment this individual cannot organize their thoughts so that they can ask the questions that will come later.

FACILITATING ABSORPTION OF BAD NEWS

A very common reaction to bad news is total disbelief. This is particularly true if there are no outward signs to reinforce the news. For example, a mother brought to an outpatients department because her child has been involved in a road traffic accident may not believe that it is her child until she sees him. If the child has been taken to theatre, or if efforts are being made to resuscitate him, then the mother may well have to sit with the news but no sense of reality for a considerable time. For this reason a debate is currently underway as to whether relatives should be allowed into the room where resuscitation is taking place. The argument for this would be that the mother would be there, would see her child, and would know exactly what was going on, which would improve her sense of reality. The argument against such practice is that it might be too upsetting for the parent. The matter was debated by the Royal College of Nursing at their annual Congress in 1997, where strong feelings erupted as a delegate gave a devastating account of how she felt when witnessing the unsuccessful attempt to resuscitate her young grandson after he had drowned. In spite of this, the vote in favour was 55%, showing a move towards meeting relatives' needs to be present during attempted resuscitation of a loved one. Hopefully, relatives will, in the future, be allowed to make an informed choice as to whether they do want to be where their loved one is even if they are fighting for life. Consider the following exchange:

Mrs Vince: Nurse, could you help me? The police told me that my son had been brought here, that he'd had an accident.

Nurse: Can you tell me your name dear?

Mrs Vince: Mrs Vince, my son's Billy, he's sixteen.

Nurse: Come and sit down, and yes, we have got your son here and he's in theatre at the moment.

Mrs Vince: Is he all right? Tell me he's all right.

Nurse: What did you understand from the police?

Mrs Vince: Well, they said that he'd come off his motorbike and he'd tangled with a car and that he was down here. They didn't say how he was.

Nurse: Well, I'm afraid he's been very seriously injured.

Mrs Vince:	What do you mean – serious?
Nurse:	Well he had an impact blow to his chest and that's the most serious damage and that's why he's in theatre at the moment.
Mrs Vince:	But he'll be all right?
Nurse:	That's the problem – we won't be sure for some time whether the doctors can save him.
Mrs Vince:	How do I know it's Billy?
Nurse:	Well, he had identification on him – that's how we now.
Mrs Vince:	I can't believe it – I can't believe it's him.

In the above exchange Mrs Vince was not ready to accept the bad news about her son's physical state. It was a particularly difficult situation in that the nurse could not for certain say how the operation would go and Mrs Vince dealt with that uncertainty by questioning whether in fact the child in theatre was her son. It is unlikely that she will accept the reality of what has happened until she has actually seen her son.

It can be seen from the above that there are difficulties in facilitating the absorption of bad news unless there is clear evidence to show that the news is correct. The capacity to absorb the news will be very individual, some people denying reality while others stoically appear to accept it. Often the bad news follows a premonition that something bad is going to happen to a loved one. In cases like this, the relative may well say, 'I knew it – I just knew there was something not quite right'. It is difficult to explain such premonitions but they do appear to help an individual to accept the reality of the bad news situation.

Occasionally an individual may have such difficulty in accepting what is being said to them that they ask to have it repeated. This can seem quite irritating to the health professional until they realize that the individual who is asking for the information yet again is attempting to convince themselves that they are hearing the news correctly. It may even be that they are so disturbed by the situation in which they find themselves that they are not hearing all the words that are being said. Again, this can be avoided by giving information at the individual's pace and being willing to stop and allow them to query what has been said.

Mr Timms: Tell me again what you're going to do.

Doctor: You mean the operation?

Mr Timms: Yes, yes, the operation.

Doctor: What did you not understand when I was explaining it to you?

Mr Timms: I don't think I understand any of it. I just can't take it in.

Doctor: Well, shall I explain it now or would you rather make some time when you're feeling a little more calm?

Mr Timms: Yes, I think that would be best. I don't think I'm going to take anything in just now.

In the above sequence Mr Timms was accepting that he was in such a state of shock that his mind could not get round the practicalities of his forthcoming operation. In facilitating the absorption of news it is important to recognize the point at which the patient or relative is suffering from information and/or emotional overload.

RECOGNIZING SHOCK

Shock can be said to occur when there is a profound physical
or mental disturbance. That bad news precipitates shock has
already been discussed but what is important is to recognize
the level of shock in which an individual finds themself and to
make sure that support is available at the time. Physically the
individual may have a lowered blood pressure, rapid heart
beat, and a subsequent loss of concentration. Those suffering
from profound shock may faint and this physical symptom
will bring immediate support and concern. What is more difficult to recognize is the level of shock where fainting does not
occur but nevertheless the individual who has heard the bad
news is disoriented at some level. For example, Mr Timms'
inability to absorb a very simple explanation of a colostomy
operation was not because he was unintelligent but because he
was too shocked to absorb the information being offered to
him. Certainly it is not uncommon for people in shock to
have no memory of that period of shock.

Nurse: You say you were asleep when we rang you
              from the hospice.

Mrs Oswald: Yes, well I'd been up with her night and day
              until she came into the hospice. I was very
              tired.

Nurse: Can you remember exactly what happened?

Mrs Oswald: Well, they phoned from the hospice to say
              she wasn't so well and would I come and I
              said what did they mean, and they said she
              was dead.

Nurse: And then?

Mrs Oswald: Well, I knew I had to get to the hospice and

it was strange really. I knew that I had to
get to the hospice, but I don't really
remember much at all. I honestly do not
remember getting to the hospice.

Nurse: And yet you must have driven yourself.

Mrs Oswald: Oh yes, yes, when it was all over and I came
outside, the car was there. I'd left the keys
in, you know. I hadn't remembered to take
them out or lock the door.

Nurse: It was a big shock to you?

Mrs Oswald: Well, yes. I knew she was dying but I hung
on to the belief that the miracle would
happen.

In the above sequence Mrs Oswald had shown no signs of shock when she had entered the hospice. The staff had in fact remarked on how calm she was. However, a nurse had asked her how she was getting home and, seeing that she looked rather bewildered, had gone with her to the hospice door and checked that she had got her car with her. The problem then was whether Mrs Oswald was fit to drive home on her own without a risk of accident.

Shock can also show itself in what appears to be unco-operative behaviour. Mrs Vince, for example, became quite belligerent while she was waiting to hear news of her son. At a later stage she apologized for her behaviour and said that she really did not know what she was doing at the time. This may sound like an excuse to tired, overwrought staff, but in fact is probably a reality in that the reaction to the shock of knowing that her child was in theatre, possibly dying, brought out an angry reaction. She may even have felt temporarily that staff were deliberately keeping her from her son, even though at a logical level she would have accepted that they had no choice.

With some individuals, in order to identify their level of shock, it may be necessary to ask them how they are feeling. The individual who faints in response to bad news is giving a clear message but for many other individuals their reaction may be so different that the only way to identify what is happening in their world is to ask them. For even in shock an individual may be concerned with following a pattern of being strong in the face of crisis.

Doctor:	This news about your problems has been quite a shock to you, hasn't it?
Mr Timms:	Well, I'm trying to come to grips with it. After all I had half an idea, didn't I.
Doctor:	But it's still hard to take on board.
Mr Timms:	Yes, I'm afraid I'm not feeling very grown up at the moment.
Doctor:	That's OK. What's important is that we get you through this and out the other side.

In the above sequence Mr Timms was near to tears because of his fears and worries about cancer and a potentially disfiguring operation but, even so, he needed permission from the doctor before he could admit that that was how he was feeling.

ENCOURAGING REACTION

The reaction of any individual to bad news will vary accord-ing to a number of factors. The personality of the individual and the way that they normally cope will be an important factor, as will the news itself. Those who are faced with unex-pected trauma or sudden death have far less time to adapt to the situation than has someone who is adapting to a life-threatening illness and an uncertain future, and yet the two have things in common in terms of society's expectations. Walter (1993) describes the taboos around death, while similar taboos exist around life-threatening illness, not only in members of the public but in health professionals themselves (Faulkner and Maguire, 1994). This backdrop of silence teaches individuals to keep their feelings to themselves and to maintain what the British call a 'stiff upper lip'. To deny the effects of life shattering information in this way does not take away the individual's feelings about any situation. Indeed, Croyle (1995) suggests that screening programmes for a number of diseases cause high anxiety and distress. When bad news is confirmed one would expect that distress to be even more profound.

The initial shock following bad news may mean that the individual receiving that news may appear to be very calm for a period of time. It is later that they may need to be encouraged to express their reactions. This encouragement may need no more than a hand on the arm or shoulder and an acknowledgement of how difficult it must be to accept the message that has been given. For others there may be the need to explore feelings and to give permission to show emotion. So often the distressed person apologizes because they are near to tears or because they feel a little faint and unsteady. The health professional's role at this point is to encourage and to acknowledge the level of distress.

Health professionals may feel that if a relative cries, that they are responsible and have perhaps said the wrong thing. In fact tears may be a sign of emotional release. Permission to cry can be very comforting in a society that prefers individuals to contain their emotions.

Mrs Clark's husband died suddenly after many years of illness. She asked to see a counsellor to gain help for her children who found it difficult to believe that their father was dead. The counsellor recognized a tension in Mrs Clark and asked her to describe the events around her husband's death. When the tears came it seemed that they would not stop. Later, Mrs Clark explained that her young brother had died some years ago and that she had felt unable to grieve because of the need to support her devastated mother. By encouraging reaction, the counsellor had allowed the release of emotion necessary for grieving to start for the loss of her husband, but also for the discharge of unfinished business over the loss of her brother.

MOBILIZING IMMEDIATE SUPPORT

Given that many people describe a blank period after they have heard bad news, it is important to make enquiries about subsequent support for the individual. A telephone call to a friend or relative can make sure that the distressed person has someone with them on the way home. Mrs Vince, for example, when told the worst possible news, i.e. that her son had died in theatre, was absolutely distraught. She was apologetic for her tears and for her subsequent anger, and it was obvious to staff that she was not fit to drive herself home. She finally agreed to a neighbour being telephoned and sat with a volunteer in the outpatients department until the neighbour arrived.

In other situations it might be appropriate to arrange transport home. Mr and Mrs Jacks were in a road traffic accident. Their car was written off and they were both brought into the outpatients department in a state of physical shock and with a number of minor injuries. It was a busy evening and their injuries were minor compared to much of the work that was going on at the time. However, the staff nurse recognized that this couple were in a state of shock, had a number of small injuries, and were having to come to grips with the fact that their car was a write-off. They were considerably comforted to have a taxi organized for them by the staff of the outpatients department.

Probably the most difficult situation is where an individual obviously needs some support following bad news but maintains that they do not need it.

Doctor: Is anyone with you this afternoon, Mr Timms? You seem very shaken up by all this.

Mr Timms: No, I'm here on my own.

Doctor: Is there someone I can phone to take you home?

Mr Timms: No, I don't need any of that. I'll manage. I came on the 50 bus, I can go home on the 50 bus.

Doctor: Are you sure because I'm quite happy to arrange transport for you?

Mr Timms: I'm not a child. I'm having to get used to this whole business but I don't need any more help, thank you.

In the above situation, Mr Timms was not being rude or difficult. What he was trying to do was to maintain control in a very difficult situation. He later described how little he remembered of his ride home on the bus. Undoubtedly he would have been better with transport to take him home but his pride was important to him and the feeling that he was in control of at least that part of his life.

PRACTICAL ISSUES

At a time when an individual is trying to absorb bad news and its implications, there are often practical issues to be handled. Mrs Vince in the outpatients department may be

asked after the death whether she wishes to see her son's body
and what steps she wants to take for the removal of that
body. If the death has been in any way suspicious, there may
be the call for a coroner's report and an inquest. If this is so,
the relative will be asked to sign the papers appropriate to
those decisions. Mrs Vince may have to identify the body of
her son while perhaps feeling too overwhelmed to want to do
it.

The same is true of the patient who is given a life-threatening diagnosis or an uncertain prognosis. The patient who
has found a lump in her breast might be asked to decide soon
after being told that she has cancer whether she would prefer
a mastectomy or a lumpectomy. She may be so overwhelmed
with her diagnosis that she is in no fit condition to make this
important decision about her future.

When possible, serious decisions resulting from a bad news
situation should be left until the individual has had time to
absorb the news. It can be argued that Mrs Vince is perhaps
not the person to identify her son's body. If she is the only
one who can do so, then it might be easier for her the following day when the news has been absorbed and she can
perhaps bring somebody with her for support. It is too easy
for the health professional, in desiring to tidy things up and
have all the paperwork straight, to lose sight of the situation
from the relative's or patient's point of view.

When practical issues have to be dealt with in the immediate aftermath of bad news, staff members should be particularly sensitive to the reactions of the recipient. Mrs Vince saw
her son to identify the body soon after his death. She had
been in a very volatile state while waiting for the results of the
operation and when she saw her son she collapsed in a faint.
While waiting for news she had pictured her son in her mind,
pale and possibly unconscious. What she had not imagined
was the damage to his face which made him almost unrecog-
nizable to her when she saw him.

When the bad news situation involves sudden death for any reason, it is valuable to ask the relative if they have met death before. This allows the health professional to give a warning of what could be expected. In Mrs Vince's case some warning of the physical damage to her son might have prepared her better for seeing the body. Similarly with disfiguring operations. Mr Timms grasped the idea that he had to have a piece of his bowel brought out on to his abdomen. By seeing pictures of what a colostomy looked like and being able to handle and examine colostomy bags, he was able to adapt to his bad news situation more readily than if he had gone to theatre knowing little of what was going to happen. In this, timing is important. Telling Mr Timms about his operation in the aftermath of the news that he had cancer had little effect because he was in shock. His education about his impending operation came at a later date when he met the specialist nurse and she was able to give him time to talk through his fears and worries.

SUMMARY

In this chapter the need for mental space, identified in Chapter 2, was further explored, along with the need to facilitate the absorption of bad news. Shock reactions and their manifestations have been explored along with the need to encourage individuals to show their feelings in response to their particular bad news situation. Acknowledgement has been made of the fact that in response to hearing bad news, an individual may not be able to concentrate immediately on matters in hand and may need support, either from staff or from friends or relatives who can be contacted. Finally, the matter has been raised of asking someone who is in the aftermath of hearing bad news to make decisions on practical issues and it has been suggested that where possible some space be given between hearing the news and making those decisions.

EXERCISE

A relative has been told of the death of his father. He appears calm and composed.

- *What are the practical issues that would concern you?*
- *What words might you use to help the relative to express his reactions?*

REFERENCES

Brewin, T. (1996) *Talking to the Relatives*, Radcliffe Publications, Abingdon.

Croyle, R. (1995) *Psychosocial Effects of Screening for Disease Prevention and Detection*, Oxford University Press, Oxford.

Faulkner, A. and Maguire, P. (1994) *Talking to Cancer Patients and Their Relatives*, Oxford University Press, Oxford.

Faulkner, A., Argent, J., Jones, A. and O'Keeffe, C. (1995) Improving the skills of doctors in giving distressing information. *Medical Education*, **29**, 303–7.

Walter, T. (1993) Modern death – taboo or not taboo, *Death, Dying and Bereavement* (eds D. Dickenson and M. Johnson), Sage Publications, London.

Williams, K. (1996) Tell it like it is. *Nursing Standard*, **11**, 2–12.

Difficult questions 4

Most people like to feel that they understand what is happening in their life. This makes it important that they search for meaning, both in the message that is coming to them from other people (Harris, 1988) and in the implications for themselves. The bad news often makes little sense to the recipient so when they have absorbed the message, a number of questions will be raised. Health professionals tend to expect these questions immediately the bad news is given, in fact it may take some time before the recipient of bad news articulates the many questions that may be buzzing around in their head. The difficulty for the health professional in answering such questions is that the answer may well contain further elements of bad news.

THE 'WHY' QUESTIONS

In an attempt to make sense of bad news, the recipient will often ask 'why?' The answer may be obvious to the health professional. For example, Mrs Vince may be asking why her son had to die and the health professional may know from the police that the accident could have been avoided. It will not help Mrs Vince to be told this but the risk is that her distress will be trivialized because she is asking questions to which there are obvious answers (Lazarus, 1985). At a logical level, Mrs Vince may be aware that her child took risks with his motorcycle but she may not be ready for some time to identify that knowledge as the reason for her son's death. Similarly with Mr Timms who is coming to grips with his cancer of the bowel. He may know at a logical level that cancer is a familial trait but emotionally he will be asking 'why me?'

A diagnosis of cancer poses problems since many cancers have no known cause. In this situation the individual who has had the bad news will continue to search for meaning and may identify reasons for his situation that are totally unrelated to his diagnosis. In a study of childhood cancer (Faulkner, Peace and O'Keefe, 1995) one father was convinced that he had caused his child's cancer and felt that he was being punished: 'Why are they picking on me again ... I had to do National Service, used my weapon ... it's God paying me back for what I had to do ... I feel guilty ... the train robbers got off lighter than what I have – they got 30 years in prison – I've got the rest of my life.' This father was having extreme difficulty in adapting to his child's cancer and had suicidal thoughts because of his guilt and imagined responsibility.

Another set of 'why' questions are those that are linked to outcomes. Mrs Vince, for example, could ask questions about why the resuscitation team were not able to save Billy's life and Miss Avery might ask questions about the chronic nature of her anaemia and, given her knowledge that iron cures anaemia, may ask why the consultant cannot offer her a cure for her particular type of anaemia.

As with breaking bad news, it is important with the 'why' questions to discover what the individual really believes and why they are asking the question (Figure 4.1). It is too easy to launch into the answer to a question only to find that the question meant something entirely different. This is exemplified in the story of the small child who was reading an old book of his father's. The father asked him if he was enjoying the book and the child replied that he did not understand what was meant by '3D'. His father immediately launched into a description of three-dimensional concepts and commen-

Fig. 4.1 Answering difficult questions

Strategy		Example
Question.	Patient:	Am I going to get over this?
Explore the meaning of the question.	Nurse:	I wonder why you are asking that now?
Gain the individual's perspective.	Patient:	Well – they have stopped the treatment – but I don't seem any better. And I'm losing weight.
Encourage further disclosure or a conclusion from the individual.	Nurse:	And what do you make of all this?
	Patient:	Well, I think my number must be up.
Check the strength of their belief.	Nurse:	And you really believe that is how it is?
	Patient:	Oh yes, and I'm right, aren't I?
Confirm and/or discuss.	Nurse:	I'm afraid you are. Do you want to talk about it?

ted that he was surprised that his son had not heard of this before. The son, looking puzzled, said, 'Can I read it to you, dad, and you'll see why I don't understand it.' What he read out was, 'Charlie bought a comic and it cost 3d' (three pence in old money).

The patient who asks, 'Why has this happened to me?' may have a number of reasons for asking the question. Until the health professional has identified those reasons and concerns, they will not be able to give an adequate answer to the question. Jarrett and Payne (1995) posed the question on nurse/patient communication of whether the patient's contribution had been neglected. One could argue that it is not so much that the patient's contribution has been neglected but that the nurse or doctor should encourage the patient to clarify those areas that are causing them concern. Consider the following conversation:

Mr Timms: What worries me is not being able to know why I've got this cancer.

Nurse: It must seem jolly unfair.

Mr Timms: Well, yes it does. I think about all the people I know who lead a lot more wicked a life than I do and they are all right.

Nurse: And ...

Mr Timms: Well, yeah, I know it's in the family but there's several of us and it's only my cousin and now me. What makes us so different from everybody else?

In the above sequence the nurse is allowing Mr Timms to work through his concerns. In this instance Mr Timms reached a point where he said to the nurse, 'I suppose it's something in my genes' and the nurse said, 'That's a very strong possibility.' In the exploration that led to this point, Mr Timms was able to offload a lot of his emotional reactions to a dreaded disease and a worrying operation.

THE 'HOW' QUESTIONS

'How' questions might be linked with a search for putting some sense into a difficult situation but they may also be linked to more practical considerations. Miss Potts, for example, who, although a knowledgeable dietician, may wonder how she is going to continue in her work with a diagnosis of diabetes. At a more emotional level, Mrs Vince may wonder how she is going to break it to the rest of the family that her son is dead. Again it is important to understand the exact nature of the question before attempting any answers. It would, for example, be easy to assume that Miss Potts, in her capacity as a dietician who often advises people with diabetes, will understand everything she needs to know about becoming an insulin dependent diabetic. By checking her concerns it is possible to give her the information she needs without her feeling that she should know the answer to this and therefore should not ask the questions. In fact, although Miss Potts had given advice to many diabetics on their diet she had never given an injection nor had she ever checked her blood sugar. She needed help on these aspects of her disease, particularly on how they would fit in with a busy workload and sometimes uncertain hours when she believed that diabetics 'lived by the clock'.

Other 'how' questions are similar to 'why' questions. 'How could this happen to me?', 'How can my son be dead?', 'How am I going to cope if he's not here?' are all questions that are searching for meaning. As with 'why' questions, it is often useful to turn the question back on to the individual to find out more about what they are thinking and what help or information they really need.

WHEN THERE ARE NO ANSWERS

The most difficult questions of all are those where there are no clear-cut answers. It was seen that with 'why' and 'how' questions, it is important to find out what it is that the individual really wants to talk about, for often they know that there are no clear-cut answers. What is important to the patient or relative is to have the opportunity to air their own thoughts on a particular subject and to check out whether their own answers are anywhere near reality.

The beliefs of individuals about their particular bad news

situation may cause problems for the health professional who does not have a definite answer but who may know logically that the conclusion expressed by the client is inaccurate. For example, the father who thought that he had caused his child's cancer by his involvement in a war was, as far as the health professional knew, quite wrong. However, there were difficulties, (a) because the health professional could not give a definite reason for the child's cancer and (b) because by the time the nurse identified the father's belief it was so firmly locked into his mind that he could not let it go. It would appear that to have a belief about cause and effect is important, even to the extent of holding on to an inaccurate belief.

What is important where there are no answers to questions about diagnosis, prognosis, or life events, is to understand how difficult it is for anyone to accept an event without a reason, as in the following exchange:

Mr Timms: What is it about me that lands me with a disease like this?

Nurse: I don't have the answer to that, but I can see that it's really upsetting for you.

Mr Timms: You can say that again. I've led a reasonable life – I keep telling everyone I haven't done anything to deserve this.

Nurse: But you're finding it very, very hard.

Mr Timms: Well, at least you seem to understand that.

In the above exchange, Mr Timms was trying to find some reason as to why he had cancer. He knew that the nurse could not give him an answer but he also recognized that she was being empathetic in identifying with his distress. On many occasions, in answering difficult questions, this is the best that can be achieved. However, the value of this should not be underestimated, because to feel that someone else understands your point of view is very important for anyone struggling with a difficult situation (Faulkner and Regnard, 1995).

UNCERTAINTY

While some difficult questions may have no answers, others may have answers that bring more bad news or that lead to uncertainty for the future. Take Mr Timms, whose bad news has been a diagnosis of cancer. The fact that he has cancer is certain, that he needs to have an operation is also certain, but his future is far from certain. There is a possibility that his cancer may spread and there is also the possibility that, although he will have a colostomy, it may or may not be a permanent fixture in his life. When he is ready to ask questions about the future, the answers will contain a considerable amount of uncertainty and Mr Timms may need ongoing help and support in order to handle this situation if he is going to adapt and have a reasonable quality of life.

How health professionals handle questions where there is an element of uncertainty in the answer is important, for the answer to such questions can aid adaptation to a difficult situation. For example:

Mr Timms: Well, when I've had this operation and I've got this thing on my front, will the cancer all have gone away?

Doctor: Well, we certainly hope so – that's the aim of the operation.

Mr Timms: But can you promise me that's how it will be?

Doctor: I wish I could, but, on the positive side, we've caught you early and we have every

hope that we will clear the problems up by
this operation.

In the above exchange Mr Timms wanted certainty but the
doctor could not give it. However, he did give the information
in a positive way while making no promises about Mr Timms'
future. Mr Timms is left hopeful but not unrealistically optimistic.

Sometimes uncertainty is in the short term rather than the
long term. When Mrs Vince arrived at the hospital, Billy was
still alive. Her uncertainty was short, sharp, and very painful,
but it can be seen that to be overoptimistic in that situation
could not have helped her given the eventual outcome. The
problem here may be in helping someone to maintain some
sense of reality when they are finding it difficult to accept that
reality. Many patients with a poor prognosis and an uncertain
future search for answers that may not be there. This was
evidenced in the rise in popularity of alternative and complementary medicines for cancer patients where there were no
further treatment options (Bagenal *et al.*, 1990). The role of
the health professional in such a situation is to remain realistic
while not taking away an individual's hope.

WHEN ANSWERS LEAD TO DISTRESS

A group of questions that are particularly difficult are those
where the answer is quite clear but contains further bad news
for the individual. For example, a patient may have adapted
to the bad news that they have had to have a serious surgical
operation. When they later start asking questions about the
future, it may be that they have to learn that the operation
did not work or did not produce the results that had been
hoped for. Similarly in the case of Mrs Vince. She may absorb
the news that her son has died and later ask questions about

what happens next, only to be told that the coroner has asked for an autopsy so that the exact cause of death can be recorded.

In both the above situations further adaptation is required and there will be further 'how' and 'why' questions, further uncertainty. Anyone can be forgiven for feeling that they have got into a situation where bad things will continue to happen. The health professional cannot take away the ongoing situation but they can, by encouraging the individual to talk through how they feel and by giving relevant information, help them to handle their distress and move towards adapting to yet another difficult situation.

QUESTIONING FAITH

In the search for meaning after bad news has been broken, a question often arises about the individual's faith. Many people, for example, will argue that because they have led reasonably good lives and regarded themselves as good Christians (or whatever their faith may be) what has happened to them does not make any sense. Questioning faith is not necessarily a separate issue; it is often integral with other difficult questions. For example, Fred, an elderly Catholic, when searching for the meaning of his terminal cancer, asked whether it could be becasue he had deliberately not fathered children but went on to say that he had been taught that if you did good, good would come to you. He felt that he had done good and yet here he was with a terminal cancer (Maguire and Faulkner, 1986).

The fact that most people who have a faith have been taught that their God will protect them can lead to a rejection of that faith when they perceive themselves to have not been protected. This is often linked with a comparison with other people who may not have a faith, are known to have committed crimes at various levels, and yet appear to be perfectly healthy and untouched by bad news. This situation can be quite daunting for health professionals, who may or may not have a strong faith of their own. The immediate temptation is to refer the individual and their concerns to a minister of religion rather than to explore the problem from the patient's perspective at the time that it is raised.

Questions of faith are often rhetorical in that the individual does not expect that anyone else can really give them the answers. What is useful is the opportunity to explore the concerns and to encourage the individual to articulate their feelings about their God and his part in the current situation. When the problems have been identified the health professional may have to agree that the questions are beyond their ability to answer and at this point it may be useful to refer the patient to a member of the clergy, while accepting that this offer may be turned down. For many patients the opportunity to get things off their chest is enough.

SPIRITUAL IMPLICATIONS

For many people religious faith and spirituality are one and the same thing. This belief can be seen to 'trivialize and diminish the true nature of spirituality' (Stoter, 1991). Spirituality is the essence of each individual and what they believe about themselves. These beliefs may include religious faith but not necessarily. When bad news is seen to be undeserved, then the individual's belief in himself may be shaken and this can result in very difficult questions. Miss Avery, at a very practical level, questioned whether her anaemia was due to a failure on her part to eat the correct diet to keep her healthy. More difficult questions can arise when the individual feels that somehow they are at fault for something that has happened entirely beyond their control.

Miss Avery can be reassured that her disease is not in any way due to poor nutrition and so her belief in herself as someone who eats a sensible diet can be maintained. It is more difficult in the case of the Catholic who deliberately avoided having a family. What to him was a sensible decision in the early years of his marriage is now, in his estimation, being questioned. Along with the question of whether the earlier behaviour is linked with the current terminal situation, there may be a shift in his belief about himself as a person. The doctor or nurse to whom he confides may well help him to put things into perspective for himself by allowing him to explore his worries and concerns. However, if that does not occur, then he may need to be referred to a priest.

Many people go through life without questioning their belief in themselves, in their God, or in the other people in their lives. The bad news situation changes this so that all that was held familiar and perhaps taken for granted is now open to question. The important aspect for the health professional is to resist the temptation to give un-realistic reassurance but rather to help the individual to work through the current situation in as positive a manner as possible.

SUMMARY

In this chapter the difficult questions that result from hearing bad news have been considered. These include questions of 'why' and 'how' as the individual searches to find some meaning in an otherwise senseless situation. It has been suggested that in all difficult questions, the emphasis should be on exploring the true meaning of the question and the issues around it, in order to help the individual who is adapt-ing to a difficult situation to make their own decisions and come to their own conclusions with the help of the health professional or another agency, such as a member of the clergy if that seems appropriate.

EXERCISE

*A dying patient asks you the question, 'What comes after –
I mean, is there a heaven – and God – St Peter, and all
that?'*

● *How do you think you would respond?*
● *How might your own beliefs affect your response?*
● *How difficult would you find this situation?*

REFERENCES

Bagenal, F., Easton, D., Harris, E. *et al.* (1990) Survival of patients with breast cancer attending Bristol Cancer Help Centre. *Lancet*, **336**, 606–10.

Faulkner, A. and Regnard, C. (1995) Handling difficult questions, in *Flow Diagrams in Advanced Cancer and Other Diseases* (eds C. Regnard and J. Hockley), Edward Arnold, London, pp. 92–6.

Faulkner, A., Peace, G. and O'Keeffe, C. (1995) *When a Child has Cancer*, Chapman & Hall, London.

Harris, W. V. (1988) *Interpretive Acts ... In Search of Meaning*, Clarendon Press, Oxford.

Jarrett, N. and Payne, S. (1995) A selective review of the literature on nurse/patient communication: has the patient's contribution been neglected? *Journal of Advanced Nursing*, **22**(1), 72–8.

Lazarus, R. S. (1985) The trivialisation of distress, in *Prevention in Health Psychology* (eds J. Rosen and L. Solomon), University Press of New England, USA.

Maguire, P. and Faulkner, A. (1986) *The Difficult Patient*, Help the Hospice video, London.

Stoter, D. (1991) Spiritual care, in *Palliative Care for People with Cancer* (eds J. Penson and R. Fisher), Edward Arnold, London, pp. 187–98.

Handling emotion 5

In many cultures, displaying emotion is seen to be a sign of weakness, particularly in men. A famous song notes the common belief that 'Big boys don't cry'. Such reserve makes it very difficult for the health professional to identify how anyone has reacted to potentially bad news. This reserve can extend through to difficult questions, which may be asked, not as filled with emotion as they often are, but as almost mechanical enquiries for practical information.

There are two difficulties here: firstly, the bottling up of feelings may affect the way an individual adapts to bad news (Greer, Morris and Pettingale, 1990); secondly, the health professional may be reluctant to explore the feelings of the patient at the point of bad news and they may miss psychological morbidity (Maguire, 1992).

The initial reactions to bad news can cover a variety of emotions ranging from shock, disbelief, through, hopefully, to final acceptance of reality. By encouraging articulation and disclosure of these emotions the health professional can aid the journey to acceptance of the bad news situation. No matter the focus of the bad news, whether it be sudden death, a fear-provoking diagnosis, or any other serious life event, three major emotions appear to be common to all. These are anger, guilt, and blame.

ANGER

To display the emotion of anger is not generally socially acceptable, even when the anger is justified. From an early age children learn that temper tantrums are not acceptable and also that showing anger in other ways such as biting and kicking are frowned upon. Anger, particularly when it does not have the opportunity for expression, can involve a rise in blood pressure, respiration and heart rate, perspiration, and release of blood sugar, all of which serve to put the individual on a war footing (Goldenson, 1984).

Most individuals receiving bad news have a sense of the situation seeming unfair. This can lead to feelings of anger which, because of the situation, often have nowhere to go. Along with learning that expressions of anger are socially unacceptable comes the knowledge that an angry response towards some subjects is taboo. This includes anger directed towards someone who has died and also anger directed towards one's God. One result of this is that the anger is refocused on to a safer subject. In healthcare, this safer subject is often the health professional.

If, in a bad news situation, anger is refocused on to health professionals it may not be done at a conscious level. The person who has heard bad news experiences the feelings of anger and looks for somewhere to put those feelings in a way that will be acceptable. Mrs Vince, for example, may direct her anger at the team who were unable to save her son's life. One could argue that because of the shock of hearing that her son has died, she is not thinking rationally. It is not uncommon in the event of death for the bereaved individual to be very angry with those who are perceived to have been in a position to prevent the death. Similarly with a fear-provoking diagnosis. If, for example, Mr Timms had been to his general practitioner with pain and problems before his diagnosis, he might be angry with the GP for not immediately identifying his cancer. He might feel too that if he had been diagnosed far earlier, then his situation might not be as serious as it now is.

It may not always be a simple matter to pick up an angry response. The individual who makes accusations against colleagues or other personnel will show anger by what he or she is saying and the tone of voice. However, because of social conditioning the individual may feel unable to express their anger and may present 'passive' anger. Here, although angry, the individual is very controlled and contained (Maguire, Faulkner and Reynard, 1995). It is useful to remember that anger, whether open or passive, may be directed at you (a) because you are the bearer of bad tidings or (b) because you are attempting to handle reactions and are seen as part of the situation that is causing the individual pain.

HANDLING ANGER

The temptation, when confronted with anger, is to soothe and reassure and, in a healthcare situation, there is also the temptation to defend the colleagues against whom anger is being inappropriately targeted. A good rule of thumb is to remember that when high emotions are involved, logic has no place. For example, to attempt to explain to Mrs Vince that the team in theatre did their best against incredible odds but could not save her son's life will have no effect on her feelings at all, except perhaps to redirect her anger at you for siding with the people with whom she is angry. The first task of handling anger is to identify what the anger is about, because until the focus of the anger has been identified, any attempts to diffuse it will fail. A second general rule is to avoid naturalizing the anger. It is too easy to look at someone like Mrs Vince and to say that anyone in her situation would be angry. 'It's only natural.'

In a study of women after mastectomy, where the aim was to train nurses to identify those women at risk of clinical anxiety and/or depression, it was found that many health professionals naturalized emotional responses and so missed diagnosing a treatable condition. One GP, in response to the district nurse's concern that a patient was clinically depressed, went into the outer office and asked the receptionist if she would be depressed if she had had to have a breast removed. When the startled woman said, 'Yes,' the GP turned on the nurse and said, 'You see, anyone who has a breast off is going to be depressed for a while. It's a natural reaction.' (Faulkner, 1984).

The angry person may need help in identifying the true focus of their anger. Because of the situation they find themselves in, they are handling the emotion rather than looking for its cause. For example:

Mrs Vince:	You said it was the *resuscitation* team – well, it doesn't seem that they know what they're doing.
Nurse:	I can see that you're angry.
Mrs Vince:	Of course I'm angry. Poor little bugger was only sixteen – it shouldn't have happened.
Nurse:	It shouldn't have happened?
Mrs Vince:	No, oh God, no!
Nurse:	Is this what your anger is really all about?
Mrs Vince:	We had such rows. I knew that he wasn't old enough for a bike but his dad sided with him. He let him have it and – God, I should have been stronger.
Nurse:	So your anger is about the fact that he had the bike?

Mrs Vince: Well, not exactly. I'm angry with me. I let
              him and his dad side up with me to get the
              bike. I could have stopped them and I didn't.

In the above sequence it will be seen that by acknowledging
the anger and attempting to find out where it was located, the
nurse moved away from the child's death to the cause of his
death which was, in Mrs Vince's eyes, the decision to allow
the boy to have a motorcycle and her failure to intervene.

It may be that the focus of anger is in a taboo area. Mr
Timms, for example, felt that his God had let him down by
allowing him to have cancer of the bowel. In order to express
his anger, he needed to know that it was all right to be angry
with his God. Mrs Vince took a long time to admit to some
of her anger being directed at her dead son because she
believed that one should not talk ill of the dead.

By giving individuals permission to express their anger
toward the appropriate focus, that anger may begin to diffuse
(Figure 5.1). Anger that is not expressed and put into words
may build up and become out of proportion to the situation.
Encouraging an individual to say what they are thinking has
the effect of getting things off their chests so that the situation
is, hopefully, put back into some sense of proportion.

GUILT

It can be seen that from the expression of anger can come
feelings of guilt. When Mrs Vince began to explore her own
anger she identified a sense of guilt within herself for not
having more strongly opposed her son having a motorcycle. It
could be argued that her anger, redirected at the resuscitation
team, was a more comfortable feeling for her than the sense of
responsibility that she felt when she thought of how she had
given in in the face of her husband's and son's demand that

Fig. 5.1 Handling anger.

Strategy	Example	
Identify anger.	Counsellor: Patient:	You seem angry? I *am* angry – the resuscitation team don't know their job.
Acknowledge/legitimize.	Counsellor:	I guess I would be angry if my son had just died.
Explore an appropriate focus.	Counsellor: Patient:	I do wonder though if all the anger belongs with the team? I should have stood up to them – him and his dad – I knew he wasn't steady enough for a bike. I was weak.
Confirm the focus of anger.	Counsellor: Patient:	Sounds like you are angry with yourself? Yes - it shouldn't have come to this – I shouldn't have shouted about your team – I'm sure they did their best.
Encourage expression of feelings.	Counsellor: Patient: (tears)	Why don't you tell me about your anger and how you feel. He was so precious – we just couldn't deny him anything.

the boy have his bike. However, in order to work through her feelings, she needed to identify that sense of guilt and responsibility.

It was seen in the discussion on the search for meaning, that individuals who cannot make sense of the bad news they are being offered may find reasons for that bad news which again will cause them intense feelings of guilt. Fred, the Catholic, who had deliberately practised birth control felt extraordinarily guilty that he had brought his cancer on himself as a punishment for his un-Catholic behaviour. Again, there is little logic in either situation. One could argue that Mrs Vince could not possibly keep her son out of danger for ever. Similarly, the tight adherence to a religious code does not automatically protect people from contracting life-threatening illnesses.

Neither of these arguments are likely to impress the people concerned. What may help is to encourage the individual to talk through the situation and to put events and their aftermath into some sort of context. If the links that the individual have made between their guilt and the bad news situation are explored, it is often obvious to the guilty party that they are being perhaps too hard on themselves and taking responsibility for that which they could not have avoided. This is a situation where, in some instances, guilt will persist, particularly if there is any justification in that guilt. Referral to a member of the clergy or an independent counsellor may be appropriate in some cases.

It can be seen that guilt can occur for a number of reasons. The most obvious is justified guilt, where there is a clear connection between the action of the individual and the resultant bad news. This, however, is relatively rare. Most people who take responsibility for a bad news situation are in fact looking for some sense in a senseless situation. The feelings of guilt that result are extremely uncomfortable. In talking through these feelings and identifying some sense of reality in which the guilt is not entirely appropriate, a more comfortable feeling may emerge. This is the feeling that someone else was to blame.

BLAME

If we stay with Mrs Vince and her son Billy's death, we can trace a line from anger directed inappropriately towards those who could not save her son and then redirected more appropriately to her own perceived weakness in allowing her son to have a motorcycle. In helping Mrs Vince to see that the decision about the motorcycle was probably appropriate at the time, her attention then has to move on to some other focus to explain the death of her son. Unfortunately in this instance, the focus was moved from herself and her weakness in not standing up to her husband and son, to blame of the husband who supported his son in the demand for a motorcycle.

It was important for the Vince family that this feeling, that somehow her husband was responsible for the child's death, was identified and discounted. Had this not happened, the aftermath of the bereavement could well have been bitterness between Mrs Vince and her husband as she blamed him for what had happened, with the potential result that he would feel that he was made a victim for the loss of his son.

As with other emotions, blame may be inappropriate. Mr Timms moved from anger with his predicament through to blaming the GP for not making an immediate diagnosis of his problem. In fact, although he had been to his GP several times in the past year, on no occasion had he mentioned his bowel problems. On the occasion that he did, the GP immediately arranged for him to have tests since he was aware of the potential diagnosis. Again, logic will not help to shift the blame. What may help is to encourage Mr Timms to talk through his relationship with his GP: how many times he had appointments and when he did in fact talk about his bowel problems. The difference here is that rather than pointing out to Mr Timms that he is being unfair on the doctor, the carer is helping Mr Timms to realize for himself that he had not disclosed his bowel problem before the time when the doctor took him seriously. He is thoughtful, and then concedes, 'I guess I did expect rather a lot and I shouldn't make him the scapegoat.' The next step is for Mr Timms to admit the true focus of his anger.

Blame may be justified in bad news situations. If this is the case, and where possible, the individual who has someone to blame should be encouraged to tell that person how they feel. This will not change the situation but it can lead to more tranquil feelings in the person who has had to hear bad news. Miss Tilly was fifty when she went to her general practitioner and asked for a full body scan to exclude cancer. Her GP pointed out that the NHS does not allow for such a service to patients. Miss Tilly went away and six months later was diagnosed with cancer of the breast. She was referred to a counsellor for help in adapting to her diagnosis. What the counsellor found was that Miss Tilly was extremely angry with her GP and blamed him for her diagnosis, arguing that had she had the body scan when she requested it, her cancer would have been diagnosed early enough to avoid a mastectomy.

The counsellor felt that she had only heard one side of the story and so suggested that Miss Tilly go back to the general practitioner and tell him what she felt. After Miss Tilly had gone the counsellor phoned the GP and appraised him of the situation. He realized that although the GP had not been wrong in denying a full body scan under the NHS, what he had done was to neglect to assess why Miss Tilly had wanted the investigation. In fact, Miss Tilly's mother had died of cancer in her fiftieth year and Miss Tilly had been convinced that she too would contract the same disease. In going back to the GP and telling him how she felt, both were able to discuss the situation. The GP took responsibility for not having listened properly and apologized. This allowed Miss Tilly to see the doctor's point of view and to understand the main point which was that six months prior to her own finding of a lump, there may have been no clinical evidence whatever that that was going to happen. Had the GP become defensive when Miss Tilly told him how she felt it would probably have increased her sense of belief that the GP was to blame and would certainly have increased her anger with him.

THE NON-JUDGEMENTAL APPROACH

It can be seen that in handling emotions there are not always clear lines between the feelings of anger, guilt, and blame. One may run into another and need to be clarified and articulated before the individual in the bad news situation can begin to come to grips with their feelings. The health professional can best help someone to work through their emotions if they can take a non-judgemental approach. This can be quite difficult in some situations and may be affected by the health professional's own beliefs and values. Let us return to Fred, who had been given a diagnosis of terminal cancer. If the health professional talking to Fred is a Catholic, they may be inclined to identify with his dilemma over birth control, or they may judge him for not observing the Church's rules. On the other hand, if the health professional is not a Catholic they may feel that the whole business of the Catholic Church's approach to contraception is unimportant. Similarly with the victims of road traffic accidents. The health professional may well have previous experience that will affect their views of the unnecessary deaths that occur.

To stand back from a situation and to handle it in a non-judgemental way is not always easy, particularly when the person receiving bad news asks for an opinion or assessment of the situation.

Mrs Vince: Have you got children?

Doctor: No, I don't have any. In fact I'm not even married at the moment.

Mrs Vince: How can you understand how I feel? How do you know what it would be like to lose someone that you love?

Doctor: You're right, I don't know what it would be

like for me but can you help me to
understand what it's like for you?

In the above sequence the doctor conceded that he had no
experience of the pain that Mrs Vince was suffering but he
asked her to help him to understand. In so doing, he gave her
the opportunity to discuss her feelings and express her anger
with the situation. He may have had his own feelings about
sixteen-year-olds who behaved a little wildly on motorcycles
but, in not making those feelings obvious and in helping
Mrs Vince to describe the situation from her perspective, he
gave a very clear indication that he was not judging Mrs
Vince or the situation in any way but was there to help her in
her grief.

Being non-judgemental does not mean that the health
professional shows no emotion. If that were the case it would
be impossible to be empathetic in life-threatening and bad
news situations. After his operation, Mr Timms had great
difficulty in looking at his colostomy. He found the whole
thing disgusting and abnormal. The nurse, aware that Mr
Timms was very unhappy, asked him if he could tell her what
his problems were.

Mr Timms: Well, look at that great blob on my stomach.
            Who's going to love me now? Look at you,
            you're the same age as my girlfriend. How
            would you feel if your boyfriend had one of
            these?

Nurse: I honestly don't know. I suppose in a way it
            wouldn't be so difficult for me because I've
            seen them before, but what about your
            girlfriend?

Mr Timms: Oh, I haven't talked to her about it, I just
            don't know how to open things up.

Nurse: Would it help if I had a word with her first?

Mr Timms   Well, I suppose it might.
(grudgingly):

In this exchange, the nurse is not passing any judgement on
how attractive Mr Timms is or is not with a colostomy. She is
admitting quite honestly that she does not know how she
would feel if her boyfriend were in a similar situation and she
is offering a positive way forward in breaking the ice with the
girlfriend before Mr Timms speaks to her about his colostomy. In adopting a non-judgemental approach, the opportunity is there for the individual to disclose fears and worries in
an atmosphere where they know that their feelings will not be
trivialized or diminished.

ADAPTATION

In handling emotions the aim is to aid adaptation to the bad
news situation. Depending on the seriousness of the news,
then the time taken to reach some level of balance and acceptance will vary. Mrs Vince, encouraged over a period of time
to talk through her feelings of anger, guilt, and blame, moved
on to an acceptance that her son's death was due to a whole
series of events which culminated in the road traffic accident.
During this period, her anger resurfaced and was directed
towards her son. This was a necessary part of her grieving as
she expressed her feelings about his daredevil approach to life
and the fact that he was putting other people, as well as
himself, into danger. By reaching the point of viewing her
son's behaviour in such a realistic light, Mrs Vince was adapting to her loss and moving on in her grief.

Unfortunately, adaptation is not always such a smooth
process. Many people who are faced with bad news, whether

in their own homes, in hospital, hospice, or the outpatients department, do not have the opportunity to talk through their fears, worries, and emotions. This may lead to maladaptive behaviour and the need for further help at a later date. Mr Timms, for example, was not so lucky. His girlfriend was doubtful about visiting him in hospital because of feelings that she had about people who were not well. She was aghast at the idea of a colostomy, in spite of the nurse's careful preparation. Mr Timms' misery over his diagnosis and body image difficulties, was compounded for the rest of his hospital stay by the silence of his girlfriend and her horror at the idea of seeing his colostomy. His emotions varied between anger with himself for the way he had handled the situation and anger with his God for the cancer. Some months after his operation he was still without a girlfriend and very nervous of starting any new relationships. He needed help from a counsellor before he could adapt to his situation and look for a positive way forward.

SUMMARY

In this chapter, the process of encouraging disclosure of emotions has been pursued by looking at the major emotions of anger, guilt and blame. It has been shown that the important point in handling anger is to identify the cause and focus of that anger and to diffuse it through helping the individual to express their feelings. Similarly with guilt, where the individual needs to identify why they feel guilty and to talk through the situation so that they can make a clear judgement of how appropriate their guilt is. In justified guilt, referral to other agencies may be appropriate. Blame has been considered as a more comfortable emotion than guilt but one that needs to, where possible, go back to the source of blame to talk through the implications.

The emotions of anger, guilt, and blame have been seen to be linked and interchangeable. The importance of a non-judgemental approach when working with the recipients of bad news has been seen to be important as an aid in helping the individual to adapt to their current situation. The process of adaptation has been considered along with the difficulties that can be experienced.

EXERCISE

What is your attitude to overt emotion?
How do you feel you could help someone to handle their emotions?

REFERENCES

Faulkner, A. (1984) Teaching non-specialist nurses assessment skills in the aftercare of mastectomy patients. Steinberg Collection, RCN, London.

Goldenson, R. (ed.) (1984) *Longman Dictionary of Psychology and Psychiatry*. Longman, London.

Greer, S., Morris, T. and Pettingale, K. (1990) Psychological response to breast cancer: effect on outcome. *Lancet*, **2**, 785–7.

Maguire, P. (1992) Improving the recognition and treatment of effective disorders in cancer patients, in *Recent Advances in Psychiatry* (ed. K. Granville Grossman), Churchill Livingstone, Edinburgh, pp. 15–30.

Maguire, P., Faulkner, A. and Regnard, C. (1995) The angry person, in *Flow Diagrams in Advanced Cancer and Other Diseases* (eds C. Regnard and J. Hockley), Edward Arnold, London.

Denial

6

Denial is a defence mechanism that allows us to cope with things that are too difficult to face at the time that they happen. Individuals vary in the level of denial that they use and this is influenced by the seriousness of the situation. At the simplest level, a large bill coming in just before the end of the month, when money is tight, may be thrown into the back of a drawer or even put into the wastepaper bin, with the argument that if those concerned really want the money they will send another statement. There is no doubt here that the bill is a reality but the individual receiving it has chosen not to accept that reality for the immediate future.

Those people who use denial on a day to day basis, in order to cope with difficulties in their life, are much more likely to use denial in bad news situations than those who confront reality from the beginning in every aspect of their lives. The opportunity to use denial in order to cope will also vary according to the situation. Mrs Vince can deny the enormity of her son's impending death as long as she has not seen him. She can bring out strong arguments that the child in theatre whose life is in the balance is not her son, that somebody has made a mistake. This can last until the point when Mrs Vince is asked to identify the body of her son. Unless she refuses point blank to go with the doctor, she is faced with a reality that no longer allows denial. However, when she gets home and falls into a fitful sleep, she may wake in the night and try to tell herself that the reality was in fact a nasty dream and she may be able to hold on to the denial of reality again for a short period.

AIDS TO DENIAL

In a number of bad news situations it is relatively easy to deny reality. In times of war, for example, individuals may receive telegrams saying that their loved one is missing, believed dead. In the absence of a body and definite proof of the death, many people may hold on to the belief that one day their loved one will come home safely. Similar situations can occur when individuals are facing a life-threatening disease and an uncertain future. Much depends here on the way the news is broken and the honesty of the individual who breaks that news.

Euphemisms such as 'a little tumour' used instead of the word 'cancer' can aid a patient in their denial that whatever their problem is, it is not life threatening. The same can be true in chronic illness in that the individual will accept the message of an illness and may accept the reality of the illness without accepting its chronic nature. Miss Avery, for example, was told that her anaemia was the type that would not go away. She was given the precise diagnosis and its chronic nature. Later, when talking to a friend, she explained that she had anaemia but that it was not her fault because it was a chronic condition. She went on to say that the doctor had told her that with the right treatment she would be cured. This partial denial allowed her to accept an otherwise very worrying diagnosis.

The above suggests that unless the news is broken clearly and the right words are used, with some proof of the event, then bad news will not be accepted by a considerable number of individuals. Such an assumption leads on to the belief that bad news is best broken baldly so that the individual knows exactly what is going on. This does not appear to be the case. In a study of childhood cancer (Faulkner, Peace and O'Keefe, 1995), parents remembered precisely how they were told the news. Even when the news was broken in a most caring way parents could still deny. One mother remembers saying to the doctor, 'You're lying to me,' when told of her child's diagnosis. Several parents in this study spoke of disbelief caused by a variety of reasons. They denied that the situation could be happening to them and some were hoping that the doctors had made a misdiagnosis.

From the above, it seems that the coping mechanism of denial can come into play in any situation but that it is easier to maintain in the absence of reality-based information and, where appropriate, supporting evidence.

DENIAL VERSUS INCOMPREHENSION

Denial is thought to be an unconscious mechanism rather than a device used by individuals to avoid reality deliberately. One could argue that Mrs Vince would not be unaware of her son's potential for an accident on his motorcycle, or indeed that Mr Timms was totally aware that cancer was a disease suffered by family members. This knowledge may not affect the denial when it occurs but it can aid adaptation at a later date.

Some bad news situations are totally incomprehensible to the people who receive them. Maggie Dalton, for example, had been married for twenty-five years. Her husband, George, was fit and well; he looked after himself, had regular exercise riding his horse and jogging round the country lanes near their home. One day when she had seen her husband off to work and was tidying up the kitchen, she saw a police car stop outside the house. It appeared that her husband had driven a short way towards the city and then turned off into a lay-by, had a massive heart attack, and died. She simply could not believe what she was being told by the policeman because her view of men who had heart attacks was of a totally different type of man – overweight, underexercised, indulgent – and her husband was none of these. Similarly with Dr Browning, who was very proud of his son's progress at university. His tutors predicted that he would get a first in his exams and thought he had a brilliant future ahead of him. He visited his parents one weekend and appeared to be perfectly normal. Yet the following morning his parents had to accept the news that he had gone from their house and deliberately drowned himself in a nearby river. In the above cases the first emotion is total and utter disbelief. Not necessarily because the bad news is too difficult to accept, but because the bad news does not in any way represent the reality of the person that was known. Here, denial and disbelief go hand in hand as the recipients of bad news search for some meaning that will make sense of an unbelievable situation.

THE COSTS OF DENIAL

What are the costs of denial? Bateman (1991) agrees that defence mechanisms, of which denial is one, play an important part in the healthy psychological functioning of all individuals, and goes on to maintain that it is their failure or their excessive or inappropriate use that leads to psychiatric symptoms.

The cost of denial in a bad news situation simply means that the time taken between denying reality and accepting what has happened delays the adaptation and necessary grief reactions to the bad news. This delay, however, can have an important effect on other individuals who are part of the situation. This can include the health professionals concerned and also the wider family circle of the individual who has heard the bad news.

In the case of Mrs Vince, had her denial been strong enough for her to refuse to identify the body in the firm belief that it was nothing to do with her, a number of people would become involved in her denial. She might go home and tell her partner that she was called to the hospital because her son has been in an accident, only to find that it was not him. Had she reacted in such a way, then one could argue that her use of denial was excessive. In the event, she did identify the body and accept reality although the denial continued to come back in an ambivalent way for some time after the death. This meant that it was difficult for her partner to get her involved in the practical matters that happen after a death and there was some question as to whether she could go to the funeral because she did not wish to accept the need for that final goodbye. In situations like this, particularly when there are emotional recriminations in the air, family relationships can be quite severely affected. One could argue that this would be the case whether or not Mrs Vince was in any form of denial. What is important here is to weigh the costs and benefits of this particular coping mechanism.

One can argue that in a bad news situation involving the death of a loved person, accepting reality is of paramount importance. This was certainly the case with Mrs Vince, where there was a body to identify and permission to be given for a post mortem. In the situation following wars, where there may be no body and no proof of death except for overwhelming circumstantial evidence, one could argue that denial could continue to be used as a coping mechanism. However, the benefits may not have outweighed the costs: for many families, the father's room was kept as a shrine, his clothes were kept, and there was no opportunity to grieve because it had not been accepted that the person was dead. The normal grieving process was delayed, often for many years, or until the death of the partner. During that time the bereaved individual was not open to new relationships (Worden, 1992).

When the bad news is about life-threatening illness, uncertainty, or a chronic disorder, one could argue that denial as a coping mechanism has a definite part to play for many patients and their families. Providing that it does not interfere with her treatment regime, Miss Avery's assertion that she will be cured one day can sustain her without any major harm to others or to herself. The same applies to a diagnosis of cancer. Many patients go through the disease trajectory, to and beyond the terminal phase, without using the word 'cancer', or without accepting that their diagnosis is of cancer. The cost here is not necessarily to the patient but to family members who may wish to complete unfinished business. Aries (1993) perceives that this denial on the part of the patient involves other people in becoming accomplices to a lie which later grows to such proportions that death is driven into secrecy. One could argue, however, that if the dying patient wishes to behave as if he or she were not dying, then that surely is their perogative given that this may be one of their last requests to those who love them. The aftermath, however, may be very difficult for the grieving relatives, who may feel that they have not had the opportunity to say goodbye or to tell the beloved how much they were loved (Help the Hospices, 1990).

Although there are some costs to others of an individual's denial, one of the features of that denial is a certain level of ambivalence. The patient who is terminally ill may seem to be in denial but may also have periods when they are fully aware of their impending death. Such behaviour may confuse those who love them and who cannot understand their loved one's changing moods. This concern can also be experienced by health professionals. It may be that one day a patient asks the nurse or doctor how long they have got and seems to absorb reality without difficulty or, indeed, surprise. There may be relief among those who are caring for the patient that they have at last adapted to the reality of their very short time remaining. It is, therefore, confusing to talk to the same patient a few days later only to be asked which of the Greek islands one would recommend for the patient's holiday when they are better. The nurse or doctor may feel very frustrated, arguing that they told the patient only the other day exactly how things were and yet now the patient is talking about holidays that can never happen. In accepting the ambivalence of denial, it becomes easier to realize that the patient may feel ready one day to talk about impending death, yet, on another, may need the illusion that life will go on and that holidays and other experiences are still waiting for them once they are better.

LOOKING FOR A WINDOW ON DENIAL

It is generally agreed that, in spite of the costs of denial to both the individual and to others around him, denial is such a strong coping mechanism that it is broken at one's peril. This argument assumes that if denial were taken away there might not be other coping mechanisms that could take its place. In situations where the cost of denial does not outweigh the benefits, one could argue that it should be left in place and no attempt made to confront the individual with reality. The opposing argument is that people need reality in order to adapt and, therefore, efforts should be made to break the denial.

A middle ground is to explore the denial and make some judgement on how solid the denial is and how important it is to the individual concerned. This is called 'looking for a window on denial' and is illustrated in the following interaction:

Mr Timms: The doctors have got it all wrong, nurse, they say that the cancer's got elsewhere but they're wrong. I'm sure that when I'm stronger, they'll be able to put me back how I was before and I'll be better then.

Nurse: You sound pretty sure.

Mr Timms: Yes, I know that I'm not too well at the moment but as soon as I get better I know that I'll be able to do things like I did before.

Nurse: Is there ever any time, even for a few moments, when you're not so sure that you'll get better?

Mr Timms: No, well sometimes – you know how it is, you get that little worry – but what if I don't?

Nurse: And how does that leave you feeling?

Mr Timms: Oh, it only lasts a little while and then I realize I'm just being silly. I'm quite an optimistic person really and I'm not too worried. It's just I'm going through a bad patch at the moment.

In the above exchange the nurse was testing the strength of Mr Timms' denial and she did find a small window of reality coming in from time to time. At this stage Mr Timms was able to push those reality thoughts from his conscious mind in order to maintain his denial of the seriousness of his situation.

Sometimes the window is larger and marks the beginning of acceptance for the individual. Mr Timms had been planning to go on holiday once he was stronger and had asked various health professionals to advise him on the best place to go. Later, however, he showed that he was beginning to get a better sense of reality and beginning to let go of his denial.

Nurse: How are things now, Mr Timms?

Mr Timms: Well, you know I was thinking of that holiday?

Nurse: Yes, you were talking about going to Malta, weren't you?

Mr Timms:	Do you think I'll get there?
Nurse:	What makes you ask me that just now?
Mr Timms:	Well, I keep telling myself I'm going to get better but it isn't happening is it?
Nurse (gently):	I'm afraid it isn't.
Mr Timms:	So, I just can't bear to think about it. I think what's going to happen and then I think I'm not pessimistic. I just wish I could get stronger.
Nurse:	And do you think you will?
Mr Timms:	Not the way I feel today.

In the above exchange Mr Timms makes clear that he is beginning to doubt his optimism and is on the road to accepting the reality of his situation, difficult though that may be.

Occasionally the denial is complete and looking for a window will bring a strong response that there is never any time when the individual doubts the positive outcome of their situation. Even here, though, the situation may change over time. The important point in looking for a window on denial is that it gives the individual the chance to review the situation without making them feel that they are forced to accept reality when they are not ready to do so.

Many relatives may want to collude with the denial (see Chapter 7) but those who are more reality-based may need to be helped to understand the function of denial, even though that denial causes problems for the rest of the family. They may need to develop the ability to interact with the patient without either buying into their denial or attempting to destroy it.

CONFRONTING REALITY

Some help may be needed in those situations where denial is not an option in any sense. Mrs Vince, for example, was very nervous when she was asked to identify her son, Billy, after his death. She needed support in deciding to do this sooner rather than later, support during the event, and some help after the event.

In a busy outpatients department, it is very easy to say the job is over when the part involving the health professional is finished. Mrs Vince was so upset by her ordeal that staff felt that she would be unable to go home alone. She elected to have a neighbour collect her who she knew would not ask the nurse any difficult questions on the telephone. When the neighbour arrived, the nurse was able to talk to her and as a result the neighbour offered to go into the house with Mrs Vince and help her to break the news that Billy was dead to her husband and other children. At Mrs Vince's request the local vicar was telephoned and told about Billy so that there would be some support at the house that would be comfortable for both Mr and Mrs Vince, who were regular churchgoers.

Confronting reality was not a simple matter for Mrs Vince but she had the strength to know that she had to see her son and accept the truth. Some individuals have considerably more difficulty in confronting reality. Mrs Morgan's son died of leukaemia at age eleven. Mrs Morgan denied the event to the extent that she would not see her son after the death, did not feel able to go to the funeral, and could not bring herself to go to the crematorium. Her denial of reality had a considerable impact on her family, for she continued to keep her son's room as if he was coming back to it and rebuffed any help that was offered. In a situation like this, the average health professional would not be able to confront this lady with her reality and she did, in fact, need to be referred for psychiatric help.

In helping an individual to confront reality, the health professional requires great sensitivity and to know when it is appropriate to refer for more specialized help if the denial is having a profound effect on the individual's ability to function in society.

SUMMARY

In this chapter, denial as a coping mechanism has been explored in the context of having difficulty in accepting a bad news situation. It has been seen that denial can protect the individual from reality and give them an opportunity to slowly adapt and accept the news. Denial is aided when there is a lack of appropriate information or evidence to support the bad news that is given.

A distinction has been made between denial and incomprehension where the individual finds it almost impossible to accept the bad news because it does not fit with their beliefs or previous knowledge of the situation. The costs of denial have been considered in balance with the benefits in situations where denial is a recognized coping mechanism. Finally, denial has been considered in terms of testing its solidity and looking for ambivalence and a move towards reality. This has been linked with situations where denial is not appropriate and the individual needs to be confronted with a very painful reality.

EXERCISE

```
0 ————————————————————————————— 10
denial                                      acceptance
```

The continuum above shows denial at one end and acceptance at the other. Taking denial as a need to avoid painful situations, put a cross on the continuum to show your probable reactions to the following:

- *A large bill arrives which you were not expecting and which you cannot currently afford to pay.*
- *A special friend indicates that they are withdrawing from their relationship with you.*
- *A loved aunt is very ill.*

For each situation:
- *If you marked 0–3, how did you rationalize?*
- *If you marked 6–10, how painful would it be?*

REFERENCES

Aries, P. (1993) Death denied, in *Death, Dying and Bereavement* (eds D. Dickenson and M. Johnson), Open University Press, London, pp. 11–16.

Bateman, A. (1991) Borderline personality disorder, in *Textbook of Psychotherapy in Psychiatric Practice* (ed. J. Holmes), Churchill Livingstone, Edinburgh, pp. 335–59.

Faulkner, A., Peace, G. and O'Keeffe, C. (1995) *When a Child has Cancer*, Chapman & Hall, London, pp. 55–75.

Help the Hospices (1990) *Child of a Dying Parent*, Screne Productions, London.

Worden, W. (1992) *Grief Counselling and Grief Therapy*, Tavistock, London.

Collusion

7

It was seen in Chapter 1 that breaking bad news is neither an easy nor an enviable task, for the human need is to leave individuals with positive messages. This is particularly true in healthcare, where professionals see themselves in a role dedicated to helping others to recover from disease. It may be even harder for a family member to know that a loved person is to hear bad news.

Collusion, that is the protecting of another from bad news, occurs for a number of reasons. The first of these is an overwhelming need to protect a loved one from potential distress. A second reason is the perceived disruption of family relationships when bad news is broken (Comaroff and Maguire, 1981). A third reason, and this occurs particularly between adults and children, is the emphasis on short-term goals, i.e. to keep an individual happy in the immediate future without thought to the long-term consequences (Faulkner, 1995).

In some bad news situations, such as disaster or sudden death, collusion is not possible, though even here family members may delay passing the bad news on to other involved people – with devastating effect. Michael was at university when his mother died. His father delayed giving him the news until after his examinations in the belief that this would somehow protect him until he was over the stress of the examinations. This type of collusion, even though it lasts a brief period, is generally motivated by short-term rather than long-term thinking. Michael did very well in his exams but his anger at his father for being denied the right to see his mother before her death, and the right to have been told when she had died, affected his ability to grieve normally and had a long-term effect on his relationship with his father. He was also angry with his mother for having colluded with his father to exclude him from both the death and the opportunity to say goodbye.

Where healthcare is concerned, the bad news situations in which collusion is most likely to occur are life-threatening illnesses, poor prognosis, and diagnosis of chronic illness. It is particularly likely to occur if relatives are given the news before the patient. The relative will argue that they know the patient best and can make the best decisions for them. However, in a large study of information needs in west Scotland (Meredith *et al.*, 1996), it was found that 79% of patients wanted as much information as possible and 96% of patients had a need or an absolute need to know if they had cancer. The conclusions were that almost all patients wanted to know their diagnosis and most wanted to know about prognosis, treatment options, and side effects. This study throws considerable doubt on the belief that optimism (a form of collusion) is an appropriate option in life-threatening diseases (Brewin, 1996).

Given that most people who express a need for collusion know the other person very well, one could argue that it is a coping mechanism that should not be disturbed. It can be further argued that if bad news is not mentioned or discussed, then a family can operate quite happily together with less stress than if the news were made available to all. Unfortunately, this does not appear to be the case. When people know each other reasonably well, they are aware by both verbal and non-verbal messages whether there are tensions and whether there is a feeling that secrets are being kept. This may lead to barriers being raised within couples and their families which make even the simplest conversation complex and difficult. If a health professional becomes involved in this situation, there is a need to assess exactly what is happening and then to attempt to work with the collusion to promote a more open dialogue between the parties concerned. This should then make it possible for goodbyes to be said and unfinished business to be resolved.

SAYING GOODBYE

Collusion is seldom the result of logical thinking. Overriding thoughts are likely to be of the here and now and of the need to put all thoughts of the bad news to one side. It is often helpful for the professional, before attempting to break collusion, to consider the overall long-term effects of the attempt to protect another from pain.

The most difficult area for the bereaved person may be the knowledge that there was no opportunity to say goodbye. This happens in sudden death, suicide, and disaster situations, where it cannot be avoided. It also happens in collusion but here, with help from the professional, it can be avoided. The bereaved individual can be very comforted by intimate conversations prior to death when each person has the opportunity to disclose feelings otherwise unspoken.

Milly had been an unwanted child, coming too soon after her brother. She sensed from an early age that she was less loved than her brother and younger sisters. Throughout her life she strived to work hard and impress her mother and so win a special place in her heart. Milly looked after her mother when she was dying but was outwardly cheerful about the future:

Milly: You are looking better today.

Mother: It isn't how I'm feeling. I think we both
          know the score.

Milly: Oh mum!

Mother: You've been a good girl Milly – and I haven't
             always been fair to you – but I'd rather have
             you here right now. I'm proud of you.

Milly: I wouldn't be anywhere else while you need me.

A simple dialogue, but Milly's bereavement was aided by the
knowledge that she had been a loved daughter. This could not
have happened if collusion had been sustained.

THE COLLUDER

The colluder will have powerful arguments as to why their
loved one should not be told the bad news and will believe
implicitly that their action is in the interest of the patient or
relative. They will argue long-term relationships, intimate
knowledge of reactions to crisis situations and perspective on
how the other person would perceive the news were they to
hear it.

In such a situation, the aim should be to work with the
colluder to open up the situation rather than to persuade them
that their perception is inaccurate and inappropriate. Figure
7.1 suggests a framework for working with the colluder
towards a more open approach. The first step is to discover
the true reasons for the request for collusion and to encourage
some further thoughts on the current situation. For example,
the relative who wants to protect her husband from finding
out that his disease is terminal may be so absorbed with the
need to protect that she has not thought that her husband
may have his own ideas of what is going on. To encourage the
colluder to articulate their thoughts in this way can bring the
opening that will allow negotiation for a dialogue with the
patient.

Fig. 7.1 Breaking collusion

Strategy	Example	
Assess the reason for the request.	Colluder:	He mustn't be told.
	Doctor:	Can you tell me *why* you don't wish him to be told?
	Colluder:	He couldn't take it – if he gets a cold he thinks he's dying.
Encourage reality.	Doctor:	But what do you think he is making of the present situation?
	Colluder:	Well, he knows he is ill …
	Doctor:	And?
	Colluder:	Yes, he is asking questions but I know he couldn't take it.
Negotiate access.	Doctor:	I'd like to talk to him – to find out what he thinks.
Promise discretion.	Doctor:	If he is unaware of the situation, and does not wish to discuss it – of course I will not pursue things. We need to work at his pace.
	Colluder:	Well, if you are sure you won't let anything drop.
Leave an opening.	Doctor:	I can promise that I will not spell things out if he doesn't want it – but if he does want to discuss his outlook, I will need to work with that.

In negotiating access it is important to promise discretion.
The relative's main fear may be that someone will clumsily tell
her husband that there is no more treatment and that he now
needs palliative care. The promise to work at the patient's
pace and to respond to his needs can be very reassuring for
the worried partner, who not only wants to keep her husband
happy, but is also fearful of his reactions when he hears the
truth.

Some relatives may find it quite difficult to articulate all the
reasons why they do not want their partner told of any bad

news, whether this is to do with diagnosis, prognosis, or treatment options. In this situation, it may help to ask the colluder to identify both the pros and cons of continuing the collusion (decision analysis). This approach leaves the colluder in control and feeling that their beliefs are respected. It is very unusual in such a situation for the colluder to find no reasons why the health professional should not talk to the patient, if only to find out his perceptions of the current situation. Here, the promise of discretion may have to extend to promising that the patient will not be given any information unless he specifically asks for it.

For the health professional, having promised discretion in order to discover the patient's perception of the current situation, it is important to leave an opening for moving towards reality. It is possible to promise not to break bad news but at the same time to leave open the option to respond to the patient's questions and perceptions.

When working with the colluder it is important to remember the cost of keeping the secret from someone much loved. This can be acknowledged by asking the colluder how hard it has been to keep the secret. While not making it explicit, this gives the opportunity for the colluder to feel a sense of relief that someone else understands them, respects their view, but is prepared to move things on without harming the patient by disclosing that which he may not wish to hear.

THE PATIENT

In assessing a patient's knowledge of their current situation it may be that they are found to be in denial and do not wish to discuss the bad news elements of their current situation. In such cases, collusion will remain complete until the patient moves from his denial to a level of acceptance of reality. In other cases, however, the patient is often well aware of what is going on. Even if they have not explored issues with the doctor or nurse, they may well, by talking to other patients, by using their own life experience, and by other methods, have a very clear idea of their outlook. They may not have discussed the situation with their loved ones for the same reasons that the loved ones have not discussed it with them. This two-way collusion is very common, particularly in the case of a life-threatening diagnosis and chronic illness. Very few patients accept an illness without making some attempt to find a reason for their current situation.

PROMOTING DISCLOSURE

Most people find it difficult to talk about death and dying. Walter (1993) considers whether this is a taboo subject, concluding that death is being identified as a new taboo, and that many dying and bereaved people already agree that it is taboo. This difficulty in talking of impending death, and indeed other bad news subjects, may be a further reason for collusion. The issues are simply seen as too difficult to raise or discuss. In the typical collusion situation, where the colluder and the patient are both trying to protect each other, the silence will not necessarily be broken when each finds that the other knows the true situation. As one patient put it, 'I would love to talk to her about what's going on – there's so many things I want to say but I just don't know where to start.'

This problem of raising a difficult subject and talking about it may necessitate some help from the health professional who is working with the family. Once the couple start talking, then the barriers will come down and the individuals concerned can begin to handle a bad news situation in an agreed and unified way. This third stage (Figure 7.2) in the process of breaking collusion, will generally need very little

Fig. 7.2 The three phases of breaking collusion.

(1) Negotiate access to the patient/relative.
     Acknowledge the cost of hiding the truth.

(2) Gain the patient's perspective/knowledge.

(3) Facilitate the couple's acknowledgement of the true situation.
     Offer support.

input from the health professional. The doctor or nurse may simply need to state the facts and then leave the couple to interact. What follows immediately may be very emotional as each individual realizes that the other has been keeping a secret. Angry words may aid emotional discharge and eventually the couple may well agree that each has been trying to protect the other and move on to what they are going to do now that they are both aware of each other's concern and able to talk about the situation.

It is a fallacy to assume that every couple share their deepest thoughts on a regular basis. In a crisis situation they may find out more about each other than they had learned in previous years. As in any bad news situation, the role of the health professional may be to pick up the pieces and help the individuals to move on to make plans, given the constraints of the particular bad news to which they are having to adjust. For the individual who is adjusting to a terminal illness and a shortened life expectancy, the issues may be to do with plans for a future in which they themself cannot take part. This can be emotionally draining on both sides, but may well aid the process of bereavement after the death, since the bereaved person will know that they have dealt with any unfinished business and that the wishes of the dead person can be carried out.

DIFFERENTIAL COPERS

In some situations, reactions to bad news may lead to collusion because of the dynamics of the relationship and the fact that family members cope very differently from each other. In this differential coping it may be that one partner is aware of their diagnosis and wants to talk about it while the other also knows but does not wish to bring matters into the open.

Personalities do not change. Mr and Mrs Earnshaw had been married for forty years when Winnie learnt that she had terminal cancer. Her husband, always a silent man, was told of his wife's disease but refused to discuss it. Winnie was desperate to talk and to begin to put her affairs in order, while her husband, coping in his usual way, behaved as if nothing had changed.

In such a situation, the health professional may not be able to promote openness since it would require too great a change on the part of one of the individuals concerned. A strategy that may ease the situation is to encourage Winnie to write her thoughts down for her husband. This helps her to discharge feelings but leaves to her husband the choice of whether to read the letter.

In fact, Winnie did write a letter and left it on her husband's desk. It was never mentioned between them but the following day Mr Earnshaw brought some flowers in from the garden and said gruffly, 'We've been OK, you and me,' before going out again. Winnie subsequently worked with her daughter to sort out her affairs.

CHILDREN

Children may be excluded from any bad news situation, both in the belief that the child will not be able to handle the situation, and with the desire to protect the child from unhappiness. If parents do decide to share bad news with children in the family, they are often unsure how to bring the subject up and when is a good time to tell a child something serious that they may not wish to know.

Mrs Archer's husband was dying. He was nursed at home and his four-year-old daughter, Jane, was a frequent visitor to his room. As Mr Archer's disease progressed and it was obvious that he would die within the next few days, Mrs Archer was advised to send Jane to her grandmother's until after the death. Jane had accepted her father's condition, had asked no questions, and therefore the matter of death had not been mentioned. When she returned from her grandmother's house after the funeral of her father, she was told that her daddy had gone to heaven. Two months later, Jane needed help for her violent behaviour towards her mother which had never, ever occurred before. When Jane was assessed by a counsellor, she made it clear that she was very angry with her mother. She believed that while she herself was at granny's, mummy had sent daddy away and would not let him come back. It needed considerable work with Jane before she could accept her father's death and her exclusion from that death. It is argued here that if Jane had stayed in the house throughout her father's illness, to and beyond the point of death, she would have better understood the sequence of events and could have been helped by witnessing and sharing the reality of her mother's grief.

The health professional's role in avoiding collusion with children is to help parents find a way to handle the situation so that it is reality-based. What most parents need to know is that telling a child that someone they love is dying is not a one-off event. Rather they should be encouraged to answer their child's questions as they arise and then, as with any bad news situation, the child will learn the truth at a pace that is controlled by them. If, for example, Jane had stayed at home during her father's last days, she could well have asked her mother why daddy was sleeping so much. This could have been the first question of many that would lead to the point where mummy would have to say to Jane that one day daddy would not wake up any more and that would be the day that he was going to heaven (or to whatever designation accords with family beliefs). This requires considerable strength from a parent already distressed by the forthcoming death, but involving the child can help the latter adapt to reality and to feel part of the situation rather than excluded from it.

If collusion has already occurred and the health professional is involved in telling the child the truth, then the process is the same as with an adult in that first of all the child should be asked to tell the story from their perspective. Often in these circumstances it transpires that the child is much better informed than their parents expect. For example:

Chris: Dad said she was going to live. I knew she was dying as one of my mate's mum had died about six weeks beforehand of the same thing, so I knew she was dying when she went back into hospital the second time, about a week before she did die, and yet everyone kept saying that she's going to live, she's going to be alright. (Help the Hospices, 1991).

Chris remained extremely angry with his father for a considerable period after his mother's death. The anger was so intense that it blocked his ability to grieve for his mother. It was a year after her death before he asked for help.

WHEN TO WITHDRAW

Although health professionals may become involved in collusion, the passing of information within and between families is not necessarily a matter for those in health care. However, if doctors and nurses are asked to collude or if they observe that collusion is occurring, then they do have a responsibility to attempt to break that collusion. The benefits of not colluding, generally, outweigh the costs but the health professional has to accept that family members make their own choices. Christopher's father would not discuss his wife's impending death with her and so he felt obliged to collude against his children in case they should tell their mother something that would bring the matter out into the open. The district nurse visited Christopher's mother one day, having talked to his father, and found that she knew that she was dying.

District nurse:	So, you know the way things are going and your husband hasn't talked to you about his feelings, I wonder whether it would help to bring things out into the open.
Pam:	No. This is the last gift I can give to Rob.
District nurse:	The last gift?
Pam:	Yes. The only way he can cope is to pretend that everything is OK and that I'm going to get better, and so he's working hard to keep things normal. I want to give him that – time enough later to talk.

The district nurse made no further attempt to break collusion within the family because she recognized that although they had not talked about it, both Rob and Pam had made informed choices as to how her death would be managed. The implications for the children were another issue, but sadly, Pam died before that issue was addressed. It is too easy to criticize parents for not involving their children in bad news situations. They need help to understand that the loss of trust resulting from lying to a child is often more devastating than the bad news itself. The parents concerned are usually dealing with their own emotions following bad news and may be in no fit state to help their children. It is here that a close family friend may be able to offer support and help. As in other issues, the health professional needs to work in a non-judgemental way, helping parents to reach the best decision for their situation, and for the family as a whole.

SUMMARY

In this chapter, the subject of collusion has been addressed in terms of both why it occurs and the cost of its continuation. Principles have been given for attempting to break collusion, both between adults and against children, in order to promote disclosure of feelings and allow families to deal with issues arising from the bad news situation. Finally, it has been accepted that the choice of what information is disclosed between family members is ultimately down to the family themselves. The role of the health professional is to promote openness as far as is possible, and to look for alternatives when this is not possible.

EXERCISE

You meet a friend. During your conversation a mutual acquaintance is mentioned and you are given some confidential information about them. Later you meet the acquaintance by chance.

- *How might your new knowledge affect the interaction?*
- *How difficult would it be to keep the secret?*
- *How might the secret change the way you feel about this acquaintance?*

REFERENCES

Brewin, T. (1996) *Relating to the Relatives*, Radcliffe Press, Abingdon.

Comaroff, J. and Maguire, P. (1981) Ambiguity and the search for meaning. Childhood leukaemia in the modern clinical context. *Social Science and Medicine*, **158**, 115–23.

Faulkner, A. (1995) *Working with Bereaved People*, Churchill Livingstone, Edinburgh, pp. 97–8.

Help the Hospices (1991) *Child of a Dying Parent*, Screne Productions, London.

Meredith, C., Symonds, P., Webster, L. *et al.* (1996) Information needs of cancer patients in west Scotland: cross-sectional survey of patients' views. *British Medical Journal*, **313**, 724–6.

Walter, T. (1993) Modern death: taboo or not taboo, in *Death, Dying and Bereavement* (eds D. Dickenson and M. Johnson), The Open University Press, London, pp. 33–44.

Hope | 8

Hope may be seen as an element in every life situation. Israel (1995) – who puts a value on moods and inward states, even those such as depression – talks of working towards hope. In many day to day situations, hope may be seen as equivalent to wish fulfilment, such as 'I hope I'll win the lottery this week' or 'I hope that I have passed my exams.' In the first situation the hope is that by chance money will be forthcoming from the lottery. In the second situation, the hope is that the work put in will have paid off or that a lack of work will not have led to examination failure.

In healthcare, hope is often used to make a distinction between good news and bad news. Mrs Vince, when told that her son had had a road traffic accident, hoped for a mistaken identity. When she later had to accept that the child in theatre struggling for his life was indeed her son, then her hope changed from mistaken identity to recovery and she sat praying that the resuscitation team would save her son's life.

A similar situation occurs in life-threatening or chronic illness. Miss Avery, for example, reinterpreted what she had been told about her diagnosis of pernicious anaemia in order to hope that the doctor would cure her. Mr Timms, with his cancer of the bowel, hoped that he would recover with no further spread of the cancer.

For the medical profession, hope may be seen in a much narrower form – the hope that a diagnosis can be made and a cure can be found for each patient. When this is not the case, then doctors may start to collude by using inappropriate reas-

surance or by failing to give the exact diagnosis and prognosis
as far as they can tell in a current situation. Such doctors
often justify their actions by stating that it is wrong to take
away hope from an individual, while others argue that every
individual deserves the truth, no matter how painful the news
is. One could argue that in bad news situations there is little
hope to be held out. However, Scanlon (1989) sees hope in
terms of the belief that good things can happen in spite of a
poor prognosis, and Penson (1991), in discussing bereavement,
sees hope as a turning point in the gradual process of adaptation towards good memories of the dead person.

REALISTIC REASSURANCE

One of the difficulties for the medical profession is the expectation from the public that the doctor will make them better.
The extent of this hope on the part of patients will depend on
a number of elements. These may include the seriousness of
their illness, their life experiences, and their religious and spiritual beliefs. For example, 'Where there is life, there is hope' is
central to Jewish teachings (Katz, 1991). Alternatively, for
some religions, what happens in life is the will of God and
therefore illness may be accepted without hope or despair. The
response from many doctors to the expectation of cure may
lead to unrealistic reassurance being given. In Faulkner and
colleagues' 1995 study, many of the doctors involved gave
overoptimistic reassurance after breaking bad news, which
could lead to unrealistic hope on the part of the patients
concerned. However, reassurance does have a place in bad
news situations as long as it is realistic and not misleading.
After her son's death, Mrs Vince told her neighbour that
although she had gone on hoping, right to the end, that her
son's life would be saved, she knew that no one had promised
her that this would occur.

Sometimes even realistic reassurance can be misinterpreted or indeed misheard by the recipient. For this reason, it is important to check an individual's understanding of bad news when it has been broken and to correct misinterpretation as far as possible, so that hope for the future is based in some sense of reality. This does not mean pushing truth at those people who do not wish to receive it, but simply clarifying that messages have been understood.

MOVING THE BOUNDARIES

Hope as a concept is not a static mechanism. In bad news situations, hope may be tempered by changing circumstances and by the adaptation of the individual to the news. This means that the boundaries of hope may move in either direction. Bereaved people, for example, often admit that at the end of a terminal illness of someone that they loved, they moved from hope of a cure, which became unrealistic, to hope for a miracle that something would happen to prevent the death. Alternately, in situations such as sudden death, the person hearing the news may move from hope that there has been a mistake and that the situation is not as described, through to realistic hope that the person who died did not suffer. Health professionals, in the information that they give, may help individuals to move the boundaries of hope from unrealistic to realistic, but accept that unrealistic hope, like denial, may be a constant feature of a particular situation. Mr Timms, for example, started his illness with the hope that he did not have cancer. When the diagnosis was made and he realized that he would have to have surgery, he then hoped that he would not get any further problems with his cancer. One could argue that the initial hope, i.e. that the bowel problems were not caused by cancer, was unrealistic, but until diagnosis it was a perfectly reasonable hope to maintain. The doctor helped Mr Timms to move his boundaries of what he was hoping for so that he could again have positive hope, i.e. that his cancer would not spread. Should Mr Timms be unfortunate and get secondaries and move into a terminal stage of illness, then the aim of the doctor might be to encourage Mr Timms to hope, not for a cure, but for a reasonable time in which to complete short-term goals.

Health professionals often complain that in bad news situations they feel helpless in that they cannot give the patient and their family hope of recovery. By helping patients to move the boundaries of hope from the global hope of a cure to realistic hope that time will be available to reach short-term goals, the doctor or nurse can feel much more positive about the help that they are giving to the patient in what might otherwise be seen as a hopeless situation. This 'empowerment' of the patient is an important element in adaptation to bad news (Herth, 1990).

Patients sometimes have hopes that appear to be unrealistic. This is particularly so in chronic disease and cancer where the individual concerned will not accept the diagnosis and prognosis that is given but will fight to maintain their health and their ability to be in control of their own lives. A good example of this is Sir Douglas Bader, who lost both legs in a flying accident in 1931 and was invalided out of the Air Force in spite of his desire to continue flying. At the beginning of the Second World War he was allowed back into the Air Force, as a pilot, and commanded the first RAF/Canadian fighter squadron, evolving tactics that contributed to victory in the Battle of Britain. He became a great pilot and set an example of fortitude and heroism which became a legend. The patient who fights their bad news diagnosis in order to maintain their own lifestyle may not appear to be so heroic, but it does take great strength of will to overcome bad news in a positive way. There is no scientific evidence that this level of hope and determination can cure otherwise incurable diseases but there does seem to be agreement that this positive attitude to bad news situations can have an effect on quality of life (Greer, Morris and Pettingale, 1979; Hanson, 1994).

SETTING SHORT-TERM GOALS

Most people, when faced with bad news about diagnosis and prognosis, will have unrealized dreams and ambitions. By setting hope into a realistic concept, energy can be put into thinking of positive ways to realize some of those ambitions. This is another area where the individual needs to be in control of what those short-term goals might be.

Christopher was forty-nine when he found that he had small cell cancer of the lung and was given a limited period to live. Eventually accepting that the bad news was correct, he asked his doctor if he felt that he would still be alive in five months time when he would be 50. The doctor said that this was highly unlikely and, when he realized that a big family party had been planned, suggested that it should be moved forward. Christopher resisted this, arguing that the date of one's birth could not be changed.

Christopher was determined to have his fiftieth birthday party as planned and set his short-term goals for that event in spite of medical advice to the contrary. Christopher was in a wheelchair when he had his birthday party and died two days later, having changed the deeds of his house into his wife's name, sold his guns because he felt that his wife would not appreciate their value, and planned his funeral service. At one level these actions caused distress to his family but, at another level, they admired his determination and appreciated his concern for their future when he would no longer be there to care for them.

Christopher's hopes were fulfilled and this can be the case for many people who are facing bad news situations. The role of the health professional is to support the individual who is setting realistic goals and to help those who need it to make those goals realistic. Little can be done when the goal might be to see the first grandchild born but if the goal is to see a much loved child married, then it may be possible to help the family to rearrange plans so that goals can be attained in a realistic time. A first step may be for the family to accept the reality of limited time, and help may be needed in this area.

Ongoing assessment will help to discover what an individual's hopes are and will also allow the professional to help them to take appropriate steps to achieve their goals. Elsie had been given the bad news that her cancer was progressing and that her remaining time was very limited. Her elder daughter was due to get married later in the year. What Elsie was hoping for was to attend the wedding but she had not told her family how poor her prognosis was; although her hope was clearly established in her mind, she was loathe to ask her daughter to change her plans. The help that Elsie needed was in sharing her bad news with her family. The daughter then spontaneously agreed to bring the wedding forward. Because Elsie was very realistic about her outlook, her hopes about her daughter's wedding were realized (Maguire and Faulkner, 1986).

In the examples given, the emphasis on positive hope helped the individuals to manage the terminal phases of their disease. Christopher stopped railing against fate once he was planning his fiftieth birthday party and Elsie's hope to attend her daughter's wedding brought about an openness within the family about her limited future and aided the daughter in making the decision to be married while her mother was still there for her.

SETTING GOALS FOR OTHERS

Bad news does not affect just one individual. Family and friends and, indeed, health professionals may observe reactions to bad news and want, themselves, to intervene to bring back a sense of purpose. They may do this by overoptimism and by attempting to set short-term goals for the individual. Although there are some exceptions, in the majority of cases such behaviour adds to the burden of the individual who is coping with a bad news situation and adds to their feelings that only they understand just how horrible life is at the present moment.

Louise and Sarah had lived together for many years, sharing a common love of dogs. They bred Jack Russell terriers on a small scale and were constantly seen at dog shows, both as exhibitors and judges. Louise had cancer which moved on to the terminal phase. Neither she nor Sarah could accept what was happening and Louise was referred to a counsellor. The counsellor was very surprised when Sarah appeared for the appointment without Louise. She explained that Louise was tired and could not come and made it clear that it was she who needed some help. Her attitude to Louise was one of 'Let's be positive, let's show the world that you aren't going to die of cancer' and she pursued this in spite of Louise's assertion that she would like to rest and stay at home more.

One short-term goal that Sarah imposed on Louise was that she should go to a national dog show and see one of their favourite Jack Russells reach championship level. On the big day, Sarah got Louise out of bed, dressed her, put her in the car in a blanket, and took her to the dog show. Louise spent a miserable day in a wheelchair trying to be cheerful for friends and colleagues that she knew, and trying to get excited about the championship. Although the dog won, Louise went home exhausted rather than satisfied. She was meeting somebody else's short-term goal which had been imposed on her, rather than her own. Sarah rang the counsellor to say that Louise had died a few days after the championship but had been very quiet and withdrawn since that day. She tentatively asked if the counsellor thought that she had done the wrong thing.

Parents often set short-term goals for children who are in a bad news situation of terminal illness. Again, no matter how well they know their child and their child's ambitions, they cannot necessarily know what is most important for that child as they face their own reality. It cannot be assumed that every child's biggest dream is to visit Disneyland.

Nicola had a brain tumour. She had surgery but the parents were told that her outlook was poor. After a while Nicola started asking questions that suggested that she was aware of how things were going. Nicola's father had the following conversation with the general practitioner:

GP: Well, how are things?

Father: Well, she's beginning to ask questions but we
           want her to look on the bright side.

GP: What do you understand about Nicola's illness?

Father: Oh, we're just ignoring what they say at the
           hospital. That's not the way we operate at all.
           They want us to take Nicola to see someone but
           none of that's necessary. We're thinking
           positively, we want her to start thinking towards
           the future.

GP: And how is Nicola reacting to that?

Father: But that's what so worrying – she's crying a lot,
           she get's very angry with us and she said the
           other day that she wished she were dead already.

In the situation described, Nicola has no opportunity whatso-ever to discuss her fears and worries because of her parents' need to think positively and to set goals for the future in a positive way. The GP offered to talk to Nicola and found out that she was well aware of the fact that she was not getting better. When asked how she saw the future, she said, 'I don't think I'll be here for very much longer but I'd like to be here a bit longer because there are one or two things I want to do.' When the GP asked what those were, they included having time to finish a story that she was writing and illustrating for her little sister and to go to the seaside just once more.

In the above case, Nicola's parents realized that their over-optimism had in fact been blocking Nicola's opportunity to discuss with them how she saw the way things were. Once they were talking to each other in a realistic way, the family holiday was brought forward, and the previous insistence of Nicola's father that she attend school for at least part of each day, in an attempt to maintain normality, was dropped in favour of giving her time to continue with her writing of which they had been unaware up to the disclosure with the GP. Nicola's parents cared deeply for her and she, in turn, tried to match their needs. Only through open dialogue could a more realistic approach be taken.

HOPELESSNESS

In bad news situations it is not always possible to see hope of anything better happening after the event. What appears to be important in this period of time is that people show some sense of understanding and compassion rather than giving advice or suggestions. The bereaved person who is advised to take a little holiday will comment that that is not what would help at the moment because the terrible feelings of loss will not go away, no matter where the individual is, and in the early days the greatest comfort may be obtained from being in familiar places where the beloved was before they died. If hope is seen as a turning point in bereavement, then that suggests that there is some internal mechanism that moves the individual from the despair of loss to the acceptance that life will go on without the beloved (Worden, 1992).

What is perhaps inspiring is that hopelessness, for the majority of individuals, seems to be a temporary feeling. A student at Manchester University took for his dissertation the value of life to geriatric patients. All had multiple diagnoses and all were seen to be terminally ill (Spence, 1984). Spence asked the patients and their formal and informal carers to put a value on the life of the individual. Both formal and informal carers felt that there was little value in the patients' lives and little hope of feeling any sense of worth. In fact, all the patients in the study had hope and felt that their lives were worthwhile. As one patient said, 'My daughter comes to see me on Sundays and I can make her laugh, and as long as I can do that life is worth living.'

If a sense of hopelessness does persist after bad news, depression may result (Figure 8.1), and needs to be identified and treated. The individual will not be able to get in touch with any positive thoughts and may feel that life is not worth living. In a minority of cases this may lead to suicidal thoughts and attempts to end life.

Alice had seen her three-year-old daughter run across the

Fig. 8.1 Recognizing depression. If three or more changes are present, screen for other signs.

Possible physical/social changes	Possible psychological changes
Careless re: clothes, home, cleanliness, nutrition	Depressed mood
	Mood swings
May choose isolation	Poor concentration
Early waking	Lacks interest in day to day activities
Reduced libido	Morbid preoccupation with death
Increased anxiety	Feelings of guilt/despair
Disengagement from family	Suicidal thoughts / feels life not worth living

road in front of an oncoming car. She blamed herself for being unable to prevent the death and could not erase the vision of the crash from her mind. She became quiet and withdrawn but no one suspected her level of hopelessness until she attempted suicide with a drugs overdose. Alice had felt that she needed to be strong for the rest of the family. She had felt unable to talk about her feelings, so they had been bottled up. She needed considerable help to adapt to the loss of her daughter and to find hope for the future without her much loved child.

In the aftermath of a bad news situation the professional needs to assess each situation to identify the return of hope and should be alert to the possibility of depression and the need for help.

SUMMARY

In this chapter, the concept of hope has been examined in terms of its place in bad news situations. It has been seen that in sudden death and bereavement, hope can be the turning point towards a future without the loved person.

The value of realistic reassurance has been considered along with the ability to move the boundaries towards a different level of hope so that a sense of reality may be maintained. This may then help an individual in the setting of short-term goals, which can be a motivator for people who are fighting a bad news situation to maintain hope.

It has been seen that setting goals for others may be inappropriate and cause problems for those who are battling against a bad news situation. Finally, hopelessness has been considered as a temporary phenomena which, if unresolved, may lead to depression. This in turn, if undetected and untreated, may lead to suicidal thoughts and attempts to end life.

EXERCISE

Outline your own definition of hope.
In what circumstances (if any) would you expect to amend your definition?
How important is the concept of hope to you personally?

REFERENCES

Faulkner, A., Argent, J., Jones, A. and O'Keeffe, C. (1995) Improving the skills of doctors in giving distressing information. *Medical Education*, **29**, 303–7.

Greer, S., Morris, T. and Pettingale, K. (1979) Psychological response to breast cancer: effect on outcome. *Lancet*, **ii**, 785–7.

Hanson, E. (1994) *Stress and the Person with Cancer*, Quay Publishing Co., Lancaster.

Herth, K. (1990) Fostering hope in terminally ill people. *Journal of Advanced Nursing*, **15**, 1250–9.

Israel, M. (1995) *Dark Victory: through Depression to Hope*, Mowbray, London.

Katz, J. (1991) Jewish perspectives on death, dying and bereavement, in *Death, Dying and Bereavement* (eds D. Dickenson and M. Johnson), Open University Press, London, pp. 199–208.

Maguire, P. and Faulkner, A. (1986) *Assessing a Dying Patient*, video, Help the Hospice.

Penson, J. (1991) Bereavement, in *Palliative Care for People with Cancer* (eds J. Penson and R. Fisher), Edward Arnold, London, pp. 207–17.

Scanlon, C. (1989) Creating a vision of hope: the challenge of palliative care. *Oncology Nurses' Forum* **16**, 491–6.

Spence, F. (1984) The value of life in geriatric patients. Unpublished MSc thesis, University of Manchester, Manchester.

Worden, J. (1992) *Grief Counselling and Grief Therapy*, Routledge, London.

Unfinished business

Bad news situations seldom occur at a convenient time. Along with the devastation that can be caused by the news are multiple factors that can add to the level of distress and to immediate reactions. There is a common assumption that bad news may bring family members together but in fact it can bring conflict (Macaskill and Monarch, 1990). The need to make sense of the bad news (Chapter 4) can lead to blame of other family members. Mrs Vince, felt both angry with her husband who had backed their child's desire for a motorcycle and anger with herself for not bringing in a mother's veto. These mixed feelings can leave individual family members in a sense of isolation rather than feeling that the family unit is drawing together in order to deal with the crisis (Black and Wood, 1989). The role of the health professional in the aftermath of bad news is to help individuals to adapt to their changed realities without building up a dependency relationship. It is a matter of current debate that this support is not available in every healthcare situation (Faulkner and Lilley, 1996).

PRACTICAL ISSUES

Most people do not live with the fear that bad news is just around the corner – bad news for themselves or for someone they love. Walter (1993), in considering the taboos around death, asks whether the taboo is to do with an event too terrible to think of or with the denial of reality. It is argued here that bad news, whether of death, disaster, or disease, is not consciously thought about until some trigger occurs to bring the thought to the conscious mind.

An illuminating exercise to be used when working with a group of health professionals is to ask how many of the group have written their will. It could be assumed that those who are working every day with fear-provoking disease, death, and uncertainty would almost certainly have thought of their own deaths but this does not appear to be the case. The results consistently show that less than half of any group, no matter their profession or status, have actually written a will. Of those that have written a will, the impetus to do so was usually a major event in their lives. Commonly described is the situation where the first child is born and the parents think about the care of their child should anything happen to them. They will then write a will setting out who they wish to be the guardian and how they wish their estate to be apportioned to protect their child's future. Another reason given for writing a will is the event of divorce, where the person left alone writes a will to ensure that their ex cannot claim any of their estate. A third reason, less common, is when an individual has a major accident, recovers, and then realizes that they should write a will in case they are less lucky in the future.

Without a will or open discussion between family members, bad news that involves the death of a loved one can raise a number of practical issues and unanswered questions in an area not previously open for discussion. This can affect bereavement and adaptation to the loss as family members grapple with the unthinkable and the unspeakable.

The same applies to the bad news of life-threatening disease. The patient may wish to deal with unfinished business but not know how to raise the issue. Family members may be loathe to raise issues such as potential death because they feel that it is not a very loving thing to do. They will argue that they do not know what to say (Buckman, 1988). The health professional may have a role here in helping to open up discussion between family members or in attempting to break collusion (Chapter 7).

TALKING TO FAMILY

There is a further common assumption that family members speak quite openly to each other about personal things. Faulkner (1984) found that after a mastectomy operation the majority of women were not able to talk to their partners about their feelings about having a breast removed, or about the effect of the operation on their sexual life. This was not necessarily because they found it difficult to talk about their traumatic surgery, but as one patient said, 'We just never talk about those sorts of things.' This finding was reflected in couple after couple who seemed often quite shocked that anyone should imagine that they ever discussed their sexual lives and how they felt about each other.

In healthcare, a wide range of issues are discussed and it becomes difficult for the health professional to remember that many of these subjects are taboo in normal social interaction. Sensitivity is required in recognizing that sharing bad news with family members may be particularly difficult for the individual who has received the news. Mrs Vince needed both her neighbour and the vicar to support her so that she could share the death of her son with her husband of many years.

When bad news involves a life-threatening disease and an uncertain future, individuals may not tell other family members because they find raising the issue so difficult. It is here that non-verbal behaviour often comes into play and requires that family members pick up the cues so that the difficult issue can be breached.

Mrs Melville knew that she was dying. She lived in a flat attached to her daughter's house and was reasonably independent. Every year she would spend a month with her elder daughter in Scotland. She considered herself a strong member of the family and asked for no special consideration from anyone. Rather than sit her daughters down and tell them what was happening, she started to tidy up her life. When her elder daughter Molly, collected her for their holiday in Scotland Mrs Melville asked her to take a picture that had been in the family for many years. Molly was shocked and said she felt that the picture belonged with her mother. However, Mrs Melville insisted the picture should go to Scotland and remain with her daughter. After other unusual behaviour, Molly asked her if there was a hidden message.

Molly:	Mother, why are you suddenly giving away your precious things?
Mrs Melville:	Well child, I want to know that they are where I intend them to be.
Molly:	Does that mean you know something that I don't?
Mrs Melville:	Look child, we all have to go one day and I am seventy-four.
Molly:	And what else is there?
Mrs Melville:	A tumour in my stomach.

In the above exchange, Mrs Melville was having difficulty in raising the subject of her terminal illness but by her giving away things that were known to be very precious to her, she alerted her family to the situation so that eventually there was an honest dialogue. This can be painful, both for the patient and their family, and many patients need help in finding ways to raise these difficult issues.

Family members may cope very differently with bad news

and this can cause further problems. Dr Browning, whose son committed suicide, went to work the following day. His wife was devastated and interpreted his behaviour as not caring about their son. In fact it was not a lack of care, simply a different way of coping with the bad news. Dr Browning's wife wanted to talk about the death to anyone who would give her the time. She wanted to go over the details, looking for something that would make sense of what had happened. Her husband, on the other hand, preferred to bury himself in his work in order to try to forget. There are many such relationships where one of the partners copes by getting on with life while the other copes by talking, discussion, and attempting to make sense of the current situation. For the health professional, it is important to assess whether such differential coping represents a change in a relationship before attempting to work with the situation.

If there are children in the family they too may cope in different ways. Some children tend, when faced with bad news, to draw into themselves for a period of time while they absorb the news and attempt to make sense of it. Others want to talk, to ask questions, and to become very involved with what is going on. When working with families it is important to accept that each family member will respond in their own unique style and that these differences do not necessarily have any bearing on how much they care about the situation that they are having to deal with.

TALKING TO FRIENDS

If it is difficult within the family to talk about bad news situations and the unfinished business that arises, talking to friends may be much more difficult unless the friend is also a confidante. On the whole, friends wish to help in times of difficulty but many people find bad news situations difficult to deal with and feel helpless in the face of the overwhelming difficulties that they see in those who are trying to adapt to bad news. In fact the wish to take away the bad news situation can get in the way of what friends can offer in times of extreme distress.

Mrs Vince's neighbour, for example, was horrified that Billy had died. She wished to support Mrs Vince and did not know how, but her major contribution was probably in not saying what she thought of Billy's behaviour on a motorcycle. Mrs Vince acknowledged the support and was very appreciative of her neighbour's willingness to drop everything for her in her hour of need. She asked nothing more and would probably never appreciate how much worse things would have been if her neighbour had spoken her mind. Similarly, a consultant whose mother died unexpectedly was overwhelmed by the cards, messages, and modest practical help he was given by colleagues. They did not diminish the death of his mother, nor yet deal with his guilt for not having spent enough time with her, but they reinforced his view of himself as a worthwhile person to whom sympathy was due.

Friends may sometimes appear to be more important than family members. They are outside the situation, they are not affected by the news to the same extent as family members, and they can often give an unbiased view of steps that an individual is planning to take to handle the bad news situation. What is generally not required from friends or others is advice. There is a risk in bad news situations of an overdose of clichés: 'Time will heal', 'One day you'll see it as for the best', and 'We all have to accept God's will.' What is more helpful is for friends to be prepared to listen and allow the person who is handling bad news to unload their feelings. In the absence of a friend who will listen, the individual may ask the health professional to take on that role and here there has to be a clear division between a friendly professional role and the role of a friend.

Many voluntary organizations offer a befriending service (Tyndall, 1993), but here again the risk is that a dependency relationship may arise rather than a helping one. Most voluntary organizations are now moving towards a counselling service that is a professional offer of help to people who are handling bad news situations. CRUSE and Help the Hospices are developing a training manual with the aim of improving the standard of preparation for bereavement volunteers.

THE UNSAID WORDS

As an individual adapts to bad news and its implications, there is often a period that can best be described as the 'if only' syndrome: 'If only we hadn't had that row the day before he died', 'If only I'd gone with him that last time and taken over the driving', 'If only I knew what he wanted me to do about the children now I'm on my own.'

'If only' applies to all ages of people who have heard bad news. Dr Browning remembered being rather scathing about his son's dress on the last day that he was there and felt that if only he had not attempted to interfere in his son's life, things might have turned out differently. Daniel, aged eight, who could not adapt to his daddy's death, felt that if only he had told his daddy how much he loved him and how much he wanted him to get better, then maybe he would not have died when he did.

Because most people do not live thinking that bad news is just around the corner, there always seems to be time to say the loving word, to undo the quarrel, or to reach better understanding. Bad news brings lost opportunities into sharp relief and engenders feelings of both guilt and remorse. When working with those who are adapting to bad news it can help enormously to encourage the individual to verbalize the words that they wished they had said. If the bad news is about impending death, then there is time for loved ones to sit by the bed and say loving goodbyes even if the patient does not appear to be conscious. After death, it may help children, particularly, to write a loving letter to the dead person, which then goes into the coffin. A more complex technique used by experienced bereavement therapists is to have a 'third chair' where the grieving individual is asked to imagine their loved one sitting so that they can say to them the words that could not be said before the death.

MOVING ON

One of the difficulties in the aftermath of bad news is the length of time that it takes for an individual to adapt, for this can be infinitely variable. Worden (1992), who writes on the adaptation to death as a bad news situation, sees four tasks for the grieving individual. These are:

(1) That the reality of the death is accepted.
(2) That the pain is felt.
(3) That there is acceptance that life goes on without the beloved.
(4) That the individual gets on with life and becomes open to new relationships.

Other authors such as Stroebe, Stroebe and Hanson (1993) talk more of a process that can vary from day to day. Such theories give markers to an individual's adaptation to their bad news situation and aids the acceptance that each individual will be different in how long they take to move from bad news, no matter its content, to adaptation to life in changed circumstances.

Chronic illness is another example of this. Miss Potts, when she was first told that she was diabetic, was very angry and railed against fate and also looked on the black side of how her life would be altered. Because of the need for control in her disease she first set about handling the practical issues and only moved on after that to adapt to changes in her life. She began to see that there were some, if only a few, advantages to the need to be very careful about her health. One could argue that adapting to a chronic disease is very much less demanding than adapting to a life-threatening illness or indeed to the death of a loved one. Each of these bad news situations brings their own problems and differing needs for adaptation. Perhaps the major difference between the bad news of death and the bad news of chronic or terminal illness is that in death there is no second chance to deal with unfinished business.

TOWARDS THE FUTURE

Once some time has elapsed, a useful indicator of how the individual is adapting to the implications of the news is to ask how they see the future. Some people are so devastated by bad news and its aftermath that they simply cannot see a future. Mrs Vince told her local vicar that she could see no point in life without her son. Mr Timms, adapting to a diagnosis of cancer, saw his future as much more short term than he would previously have believed. One could hope, with time, that both these views would move in a more positive direction. Mrs Vince moved from hopelessness and despair to an uneasy acceptance of her changed circumstances. Indeed, she felt guilty when, some weeks after her son's death, she found herself humming along to a radio programme. As she explained, 'I don't know how I could ever be relaxed enough to sing when he is so recently taken from me.' Mr Timms, however, did not change his pessimistic view of the future but he did take a more positive attitude to what he was going to do in the immediate time that he did have.

Many women have to accept the reality that their much loved baby will be stillborn or may die shortly after birth. At the time that they hear the news it is almost impossible to think ahead to trying again. Often, after the event, they will complain about the well-meaning friends and relatives who told them that they were young enough to have another baby. As they adapt to their loss, they may, at some point in the future, decide to try for a baby again, not to replace the dead child, but because they have worked through the trauma and felt it worthwhile to trust that their previous bad news situation will not be repeated. In Worden's (1992) terms, the couple have adapted to a point where they can be open to forming a new relationship with another child.

There are some people who do not move on from their particular loss. Mrs Yates had to accept the bad news that her husband had left her for another woman. She was convinced that one day he would come home and all would be forgiven. Twenty years later when she was dying of cancer, her final words to the nurse were, 'Will he get here in time?' During those years Mrs Yates had brought up her family, seen them married, and become a doting grandmother. To the outside world she appeared a happy and contented woman but she had never been open to new relationships and had lived with the unrealistic hope that her husband would return. Such cases are rarely identified but they raise the question of how much help should be offered to those who are finding it almost impossible to adapt to the reality of bad news.

SUMMARY

In this chapter the fact that bad news almost always comes at an inopportune time has been considered, in terms of both the practical issues when another person's wishes are unknown and the emotional issues around talking to other people about the bad news. The health professional's role has been explored in helping individuals to deal with unfinished business and a distinction made between being a friendly professional and a befriender. Markers have been given to assess an individual's adaptation to bad news in terms both of acceptance and of movement towards a future that is irreversibly changed by the individual's reactions to their situation.

EXERCISE

Imagine that you are caught in a 'time warp' where you may not be able to return to those you love.

- *What would you have wanted to discuss with loved ones if you had known that you may not see them again?*
- *Is there any one thing you would have wanted to do?*
- *Are there any special messages you would wish to leave?*

On reflection, what have you learned from this exercise which might help you with your work?

REFERENCES

Black, D. and Wood, D. (1989) Family therapy and life-threatening illness in children or parents. *Palliative Medicine*, **3**, 113–18.

Buckman, R. (1988) *I Don't Know What to Say*, Papermac, Macmillan, London.

Faulkner, A. (1984) Teaching non-specialist nurses to assess patients after mastectomy. Unpublished PhD thesis, Steinberg Collection, RCN, London.

Faulkner, A. and Lilley, R. (1996) *Bereavement: A Management Checklist*, Mediprint Publishing, Sheffield.

Macaskill, A. and Monarch, J. (1990) Coping with childhood cancer: the case for long-term counselling help for patients and their families. *British Journal of Guidance and Counselling*, **18**(1), 13–26.

Stroebe, M., Stroebe, W. and Hanson, R. (1993) *Handbook of Bereavement*, Cambridge University Press, Cambridge.

Tyndall, N. (1993) *Counselling in the Voluntary Sector*, Open University Press, London.

Walter, T. (1993) Modern death: taboo or not taboo? in *Death, Dying and Bereavement* (eds D. Dickenson and M. Johnson), Open University Press, London.

Worden, J. (1992) *Grief Counselling and Grief Therapy*, Springer Publishing, Cambridge University Press, Cambridge.

Breaking bad news is but one part of clinical reality for those in the caring professions. It may be seen to conflict with the notion of caring, especially in a busy accident and emergency department where bad news situations are common in an atmosphere where patients and relatives look for reassurance that all will be well. The same applies in oncology, terminal care, and other areas where a cure cannot be promised or where death is likely to occur. Such work is known to be emotionally draining (Maslach, 1981).

THE VALUE OF SHOOTING THE MESSENGER

Giving the messenger the responsibility for the words that he carries, as believed by the Greeks who killed the messenger, still holds in healthcare. Mrs Jenkins had looked after her husband through a long and protracted illness. As he became less able to get out of bed and care for himself, he became more demanding and Mrs Jenkins became extremely tired. A district nurse advised her to allow her husband to go to the local hospice for a few days so that she could have a rest. Mrs Jenkins reluctantly agreed and began to think of things that she might do, like having a real long sleep, going to the hairdressers, and visiting friends.

Unfortunately, Mr Jenkins died within twelve hours of reaching the hospice. Mrs Jenkins blamed the doctor who informed her of the death and accused him of killing her husband, maintaining 'He was all right while I was looking after him.' It is common in such cases to become defensive and to point out, in a logical way, how the hospice staff did their best and could not have foreseen the sudden death of Mr Jenkins. The relative however, may be very upset and resistant to such reasoning. It is always more useful to try to identify the underlying cause of such anger.

> Doctor: I can see how upset you are and I can understand that, but I wonder why you are so angry?
>
> Mrs Jenkins: If I'd kept him at home he would have still been there now. He would have been all right. You killed him.
>
> Doctor: Do you really believe that?
>
> Mrs Jenkins: You just don't understand – I'd promised him he'd die at home. [She starts weeping]

In the above sequence, rather than being defensive about the care that had been given to Mr Jenkins, the doctor explored his wife's feelings and found that the underlying anger was directed at herself for her perceived neglect in allowing her husband to make the trip to the hospice.

Projection is a natural defence mechanism which allows the individual to blame others for perceived personal failures or to move responsibility to another person. In bad news situations, projection can be a useful coping mechanism in the short term, for it allows the first emotions to be expressed without personal guilt being added to the burden. If these feelings are later explored and articulated, the true situation can be examined in a supportive way.

Mrs Vince, whose son, Billy, died after a road traffic accident, took many months before she could look at the situation and realize that Billy, not unlike other youngsters, had been a bit of a tearaway on his motorcycle. Had she had to face that knowledge at the time that she was facing his death, it might have been just too overwhelming. It was much safer to verbally attack the doctors who had been unable to save his life.

An understanding of the function of projection can help health professionals to see that generally, the attack is not aimed at them personally, but at them as the messenger of bad news. Such knowledge may not make these verbal attacks any easier to bear but it can help to avoid a defensive response. Acknowledging the censure, while attempting to explore the true focus of the anger and distress, can help an individual to accept their true feelings in a relatively safe environment.

DISPLACED EMOTIONS

Any of the emotions shown as a response to bad news may be projected on to the health professional. The skilled professional will not react to the responses but will help the individual to refocus the emotions in a more appropriate place. This can be a painful and draining experience for someone who has not wanted to break bad news and feels helpless in not being able to change the situation or make things better. What the professional is giving in these situations is permission for the negative emotion to be refocused without judgement as to whether the refocusing is appropriate. Mrs Vince had a long way to move in order to see that no outsider was to blame for her son's death. Her first reaction when she accepted that her son was in theatre was anger that those who called themselves the resuscitation team could not resuscitate her son. When she was asked to refocus her anger she moved on to blaming her husband and then feeling guilty that she had not intervened to prevent Billy having his motorcycle. She then blamed God for taking a young lad simply because he was behaving in an irresponsible way. Finally she worked through to the fact that there was no one to blame for Billy's death and that ultimately he was responsible for his own behaviour. Only then could she experience any feelings of sympathy for the family in the car that had collided with Billy.

As Mrs Vince moved through a variety of refocused feelings, the main help that she received was that nobody judged her for what she was thinking. Each step was accepted as a step along the way to acceptance of reality. Any attempt in the early days after Billy's death to make Billy responsible for the accident would have made Mrs Vince more angry and perhaps unable to move on to her final acceptance.

Not all those who have to accept bad news do reach a sense of reality. They may get stuck in a particular line of thinking and refuse to be moved from that point. One of the difficulties for health professionals is that they cannot always follow the story through to its conclusion. The people on duty in the accident and emergency department on the night that Billy Vince died were not the people who helped her move through the painful business of accepting her son as he really was, to the point where she no longer held others responsible for his death. Real life, too, has many complexities that will not all be known to the health professional. This may add to the strain on those who work with patients and relatives, and lead to feelings of frustration when a situation appears to be unresolved.

Mr Haws was dying and was obviously very afraid. The nurse responsible for his care attempted to explore his fear without success. As he became more ill he refused to lie down in bed in case he died in his sleep. He died sitting upright in a chair, refusing to see his wife or children.

The nurse did not forget the patient or her perceived failure to identify his needs. She heard, some years later, that the patient's wife had discovered a letter after his death which

showed that her husband had had a brief homosexual relationship. His fear of retribution from his God had caused his
fear of dying, for he was very religious. This new knowledge
of the patient closed the case for the nurse, though she still
felt that she should have been able to gain his confidence. She
needed help to accept her limitations.

SELF-AWARENESS

Breaking bad news and handling its aftermath, which may
include the projection of a range of emotions, can be very
demanding and requires that those who are involved in this
area should know something about themselves and their own
limitations. It is a common fallacy that those in the helping
professions can see every individual in the same kindly light
and accurately identify all their problems, but this is expecting
more than is reasonable from any human being.

Each individual carries baggage built from their own life
experiences. Much of this may exist at an unconscious level
and only come to light when triggered by a similar experience.
One could argue that the job has to be done and that there is
no room for personal preference. Although this is true in
general, there are specific experiences where it might be sensible to take some time out or to move to a different area for a
period of time. For example, for any health professional
recently bereaved, there should be a period of space where
they do not have to work with dying patients. This is because
their own experience may colour the way they perform and
because the experiences they meet on a day to day basis may
reactivate the emotional responses which they are currently
attempting to handle.

Although life experiences in common can get in the way of
helping people to handle their bad news situations, they can
also be helpful and aid understanding and empathy. Miss

Potts, after she had her diagnosis of diabetes and had become used to a new regime in her life, found that, she was far more empathetic with newly diagnosed diabetic patients. She found that because she had had to struggle with the issues, the control, the daily injections, she was much more positive about other people in the same situation. After a time, however, she found that talking to patients with diabetes about their problems began to interfere with her own stability about the disease. She admitted to a colleague that she felt that her whole life was dominated by diabetes. 'It's silly but when I wake up in the morning the first thing I think about is my blood sugar and my injection and eating the right sort of breakfast. Then I go to work and it seems that half the patients at least that I'm working with are diabetics with the same sort of problems that I have, and then when I come home from work at night I've got to start thinking about my evening meal, what I'm going to do socially and where that leaves me with my injections, and frankly by the time I'm in bed I feel that I've just been smothered by diabetes all day.'

Miss Potts was well aware of what the strain of handling her own disease and working in a similar area was doing to her. Her self-awareness allowed her to negotiate some time out (Faulkner and Maguire, 1994) and to reorganize her patient load with a colleague so that during the day she was dealing with issues other than those of diabetic patients.

Self-awareness is aided by each individual recognizing their own attitudes and beliefs. Rachel, as a school nurse, was being asked how she dealt with a number of bad news situations with school children. She was asked how she would handle the fourteen-year-old who came into her office, burst into tears, and said, 'Miss, I'm pregnant and I don't know what to do.' Rachel gave a wry smile and replied, 'I'd send her to a collea-gue. I get so cross with the silly children who get themselves into that situation that I know that I can't help them.'

Such an approach may seem very hard but in fact Rachel

was being honest about her own limitations and how they were affected by her own principles and beliefs. That prejudice should not get in the way of good practice is a basic principle but knowing something about one's personal prejudice and belief can avoid difficult situations for both the bearer and the receiver of bad news.

SURVIVAL STRATEGIES

The cost of caring is well documented (Burnard, 1991; Barden, 1991; Faulkner and Maguire, 1988). In spite of this there is still a commonly held belief that those in health care and situations where bad news is common should be prepared to give unstintingly without counting the cost. What each professional needs to do is to work out their own strategies for coping with difficult situations and to set their own limits for competent practice.

HONESTY

Everyday life can appear to be pretty competitive from early childhood. There is the learned belief that being best is the ultimate goal. In healthcare this competitiveness can be translated into checking who works the longest hours and who gives most to the institution. What is most important is that each individual gives the best that is possible for them and is prepared to state quite honestly when further effort is simply not possible. Most health professionals, because they are committed to their jobs, find it incredibly difficult to say 'no' (Smith, 1980). They may be fearful that in saying 'no' they are showing a lack of care. In reality they are being honest in admitting that they have no reserves left to give more to patient care.

CUT-OFF POINTS

In the Air Force there is an expression called 'closing the hangar door', which is a crude way of saying that work is over for the day. For those who are working in situations where bad news is part and parcel of everyday life, there need to be clear cut-off points to allow mental relaxation. An interesting exercise is to sit in a staff canteen or lounge. Almost inevitably the conversations are about work, about situations that have arisen or may arise, about patients and their families, and the general problems of day to day working. This means that although the staff are having coffee, they are not having a break. It is quite useful to set a 'close the hangar door' policy for break times so that work will not be discussed, and the time may be used for social relaxation.

An even more important cut-off point is the end of the working day, where it is essential to make a distinction between the work place and home. Those who wear a uniform can aid this distinction by changing into their own clothes at the end of the working day. Many health professionals report that they bathe or shower when they get home in order to 'wash the cares of the day' away. On one workshop, a senior consultant admitted that he made the break from work to home each evening by having a deep bubble bath and at the same time a large gin and tonic. Many would argue that it is not easy in demanding work to leave work behind at the end of the day. They would argue that, if you are truly caring about patients and relatives, things that have affected you may stay with you. The reality is that sometimes a particularly worrying case may leave its mark so that thoughts stay with the professional as they go from work to home. Hence the need for other strategies to reinforce the cut-off from work to play.

DIVERSIONS

The diversions used by health professionals to put time off into proportion are many and varied. Some people are helped by physical exertion such as walking, jogging, swimming, and other physical exercise. Others prefer less energetic pursuits such as watching television, doing embroidery, reading, and other creative hobbies. Yet others include animals in their relaxation, whether it be taking the dog for a walk, feeding the chickens, or riding a horse. They describe the sense of comradeship possible when working with animals and being close to nature. What is important in all these diversions is that they represent a method of unwinding that suits the individual. Such pursuits will not take problems away but they will give important breathing space while the brain may go on working at an almost unconscious level towards resolutions of the problems that have been left behind. It is not uncommon to hear a health professional say, 'I thought I'd put it quite out of my mind, yet when I woke up the next morning the answer was there. I wonder why I didn't see it before.'

The role of family and friends may also be important in presenting diversions to mark cut-off points from work to play. One problem that can occur is when the health professional expects a friend or partner to listen to their problems. Such help may not always be readily forthcoming for a number of reasons and it should be possible to make a distinction between diversion as an aid to cutting off and the need to discuss problems. In the latter situation, supervision is a better option, although this is not always available in the helping professions (Hawkins and Shohet, 1990).

TALKING

The value of sharing problems and discharging emotions cannot be underestimated. Supervision allows for work issues to be reviewed and discussed in a relatively safe environment. If this is not available as an option, alternatives should be considered, particularly if family and/or friendship support is not readily available.

Team meetings may give an opportunity to share cases and consider ways to improve practice. Such meetings, however, may not provide an appropriate arena for reflection and personal growth as is found in supervision. Some hospitals provide a counselling service for staff but if this is not available, private arrangements may be made with a trusted colleague to give each other time to offload and review work experiences.

HUMOUR

Humour can aid survival for the messenger and may be therapeutic for some patients (Lieber, 1986; Erdman, 1991). A distinction needs to be made between humour that can lighten a situation and humour that can be cruel and damaging. Humour links with self-awareness in that those who can develop insight can learn to laugh at themselves with others as a form of release from tensions.

Humour, however, is more than laughter, which is seldom appropriate in bad news situations. It may incorporate positive attitudes, patience, and a willingness to adapt in difficult situations, so reducing stress. Using humour as a survival strategy may also help the recipients of bad news, who may feel comforted by the lack of tension in the health professional, and the perceived warmth and care that are generated by good humour.

REWARDS

Rewards may help survival in healthcare. Such rewards need not be large but can give a sense of pleasure after a heavy working day. An oncology nurse was heard to say that when the going got rough in her job she would go out and spend money. This is not always possible but other means of gaining pleasure at the end of the day include buying chocolate, having an end of the day drink, having a luxurious beauty makeover, and other small treats that are seen as indulgence.

Rewards may come from outside and not involve spending money. Feedback from patients and relatives can be very rewarding when it is spontaneously given. It is suggested here that such feedback could equally come from colleagues. In our culture, it is more common to tell colleagues when things have gone wrong than to give them positive feedback when things have gone well. A change in attitude in this respect could aid survival in a difficult working environment (Faulkner, 1996).

SUMMARY

In this chapter, the need of individuals who have heard bad news to strike out against the messenger has been considered along with the need to understand that such attacks are seldom meant at a personal level. The value of developing self-awareness has been explored as a mechanism both to learn about one's strengths and limitations and to develop ways to use this knowledge to improve the care given to those who have to receive bad news. Self-awareness includes the knowledge that each of us carries baggage that can trigger unexpected reactions in the face of traumatic situations.

Finally, survival strategies have been considered that will allow the health professional to take adequate rest from the considerable demands, both mental and physical, of working with people who are having to hear and adapt to bad news.

EXERCISE

What steps would you take in the face of anger from a patient, client, or relative?
How do you think you might feel after the exchange?
What helps you to switch off from work to home?

REFERENCES

Barden, V. (1991) *Caring for the carers*, Mercia Publications, London.

Burnard, P. (1991) Beyond burnout. *Nursing Standard*, **5**(43), 46–8.

Erdman, L. (1991) Laughter therapy for patients with cancer. *Oncology Nursing Forum*, **18**(8), 1359–63.

Faulkner, A. and Maguire, P. (1988) The need for support. *Nursing*, **5**(28), 1010–12.

Faulkner, A. and Maguire, P. (1994) Talking to cancer patients and their relatives. *Oxford University Press*, 156–68.

Faulkner, A. (1996) Care of oncology patients: caring for the carers. *Complementary Therapies in Nursing and Midwifery*, **2**, 59–61.

Hawkins, P. and Shohet, R. (1990) *Supervision in the Helping Professions*, Open University Press, Buckingham.

Lieber, D. (1986) Laughter and humour in critical care. *Dimensions of Critical Care Nursing*, **5**, 162–70.

Maslach, C. (1981) *Burnout: The cost of caring*. Prentice Hall, Englewood Cliffs, New Jersey.

Smith, P. (1980) *When I Say No I Feel Guilty*, Penguin, London.

Summary

In previous chapters it has been accepted that breaking bad news is difficult for most health professionals and requires a skilled approach in order to convey the message in a way that can be absorbed by the recipient with minimum trauma. The issues of who should give bad news and how it should be given have been a thread through all the chapters, and the issue of how much bad news should be given at any one time has also been addressed.

THE MODEL

The model used in the text is based on the belief that few people come into a bad news situation with absolutely no idea of what is about to be conveyed. One of the examples used throughout has been a man who guessed that his problems might be linked to his family record of cancer. This fore-knowledge of the possibility of bad news is used as the starting point in giving the message, for it is accepted that few people who are dealing with an acute or chronic illness have no idea whatsoever as to what might be their problem. Their own life experiences or those of acquaintances or, indeed, knowledge gained from the media all help an individual to make sense of a current situation and set the scene before a health professional has to impart bad news.

For those recipients of bad news who have had no time to identify the potential for their changed situation, it has been suggested that a warning should always precede bad news. This warning may be verbal, as with the doctor who has to tell a patient that the result of their investigations show serious illness, or may be non-verbal, as in a situation where a policeman calls at a house and his uniform alone is enough to warn the occupant that the message that is brought will contain bad news.

A central belief throughout is that the recipient of bad news is in the best position to indicate how much news he can absorb at any one time. For patients who are learning about diagnosis and prognosis, this is particularly important, for if too much information is given before the recipient is ready for that information, then little is likely to be absorbed and the patient may go into denial.

The thinking behind the model stresses the need for the recipient of bad news to have time to absorb that news before being given further information. Again, control should be with the individual, who will determine for themselves when they are ready to ask questions and perhaps be ready for more detailed information.

The final step in the model is to help the recipient to adapt to the news and to pick up the pieces of their mental distress. This stage may include difficult questions, a variety of emotions, and, occasionally, unrealistic expectations of the way forward.

ADAPTING THE MODEL

Breaking bad news in the way described is particularly effective when the news involves diagnosis and prognosis, particularly in life-threatening illness and chronic illness. Here the recipients of bad news may have some time in order to adapt. It is not always crucial that all information is given immediately. One of the case studies described in previous chapters was of a patient who was quite able to accept that she was anaemic. It took much longer to accept the whole of the message which told her that her anaemia constituted a chronic disease.

One of the criticisms of giving bad news at a pace dictated by the recipient is that there is not always time when the message must be given in its entirety. It is argued here that the same steps can be taken to break the bad news effectively but that the time between each stage will have to be compressed. An example has been given of a mother who had to accept that her child had had a fatal road traffic accident and died very soon after being admitted to hospital. She had received her warning of bad news from the police, but after a period at the hospital she had very little time to accept the fact that her son was fighting for his life in theatre and that he died soon after her arrival.

There would have been even less time had her son been dead on arrival but again, the same steps can be taken in such a case, so that the first message is a warning and the subsequent elements of the message are given in stages, albeit in a very short period of time. Even here the warning that something serious has happened to Mrs Vince's son allows her to come to the conclusion very rapidly that he may have had an accident on his motorcycle. It has been argued throughout that this approach is much more acceptable than bluntly giving a bad news message without prior warning. The adaptation of the model to collapse the time required to break bad news should not affect its impact on the recipient.

In situations such as suicide or trauma it is even more important to give a warning and to allow some time for the message to be accepted. Again it is very common for the recipient of bad news, having received the warning, to make an accurate guess as to what the message may be about.

It can be seen that the time frame of breaking bad news may be very variable, but even when timing has to be adapted for a particular situation, the level of shock following bad news cannot be underestimated, nor can it be assessed until the recipient has heard the news. The relative who is expecting a loved one to die may be perceived as likely to be less shocked than the mother who hears that her son has had a major road traffic accident. In general terms this may be a correct assumption but there should always be a check made, for many people who are apparently expecting bad news are quietly hoping for a miracle and are not as far on in their acceptance of what is going to happen as might be expected.

DIFFICULT QUESTIONS

Throughout the preceding chapters it has been seen that no matter the bad news message and whether or not it was expected, the acceptance of reality may be followed by some very difficult questions. These may be difficult because the answers constitute further bad news, as with the patient who may accept the fear-provoking diagnosis of cancer. In answer to subsequent questions this patient is faced with the uncertainty that lies ahead and the inability of staff to promise a cure. When the news is unexpected, difficult questions may still follow, such as that given in the example of the mother whose son had a motorcycle accident; she had to move from accepting that it was her son in theatre to accepting that he was dead, and then to concerning herself with the 'how' of his death. Each of her questions was answered with, from her perspective, further bad news, because what she had wanted to hear was that her son would recover. When she had to accept that he would not recover, she wanted to hear that he was an innocent victim in the accident.

Sometimes difficult questions are seen to be difficult because there are no clear-cut answers. The health professional may not have the information that is required, and may have to make this explicit. Such situations can extend the trauma of bad news for those who are attempting to make some sense of what is happening to them or to their loved ones.

Difficult questions may also be linked to the individual's religious beliefs and spiritual beliefs. This can be a particularly difficult area for the health professional, especially if the current situation is shaking an individual's belief in themselves or in their God. Such questions may be rhetorical, the individual not expecting any specific answer but needing to explore feelings around the difficulty in which they are currently placed. The health professional needs to adapt to the knowledge that there is not always an answer, but there is value in helping people to articulate their concerns.

EMOTIONAL RESPONSES

Three major emotional responses have been considered as potential reactions to bad news: anger, guilt, and blame. Many individuals do not make their emotional responses explicit. They may feel that it is not socially acceptable to express feelings of anger and guilt, particularly. Along with the belief that it is a weakness to shed tears, the health professional may find it difficult to encourage the individual to disclose their feelings and to express their true responses to a bad news message.

In handling emotional responses the aim is to encourage the disclosure of feelings and to diffuse those feelings where possible. Anger and blame may be inappropriately focused, so a further aim is to identify the correct focus so that the feelings can be diffused. This requires that the health professional takes a non-judgemental approach to the individual who is struggling to come to grips with bad news and may appear to be making a personal attack. Logic will have little place in this area but, with help, the individual will work through to more appropriate responses and more focused comment.

In disclosing feelings and refocusing inappropriate feelings, the individual will, hopefully, move on to adapt to the bad news message and accept its reality. This may take much longer for some people than for others and will depend on the complexity of the bad news and the level of previous expectation of that bad news.

DENIAL

Denial is a coping mechanism used in day to day life to defend oneself against bad news at any level for a short period of time. In serious bad news situations, denial should be explored to see whether it is an ambivalent state or whether the individual simply cannot move on to accept reality.

A comparison has been made between denial of a known fact and incomprehension of that fact, and it has been seen that if there is little evidence for bad news, it is very likely that the individual receiving that news may have difficulty in comprehending how the situation being described could possibly have happened. This is different from denial where the information has been given and the receiver simply refuses to believe what has been said. Denial too can be aided by lack of evidence.

It has been suggested that, although it may be inappropriate to move someone on from denial, it is appropriate to look for a window on that denial to find out if at any time the individual comes close to some level of reality, even if only briefly. This will show that the denial is a coping mechanism for a period of time rather than a block to knowledge that is resisted. While denial exists it is difficult to confront reality and an individual may be stuck with a belief that not only avoids reality but also blocks any level of acceptance. After a death, for example, such denial can lead to the dead individual's room being kept as a shrine even if other family members are crowded into too small a space.

COLLUSION

Collusion, that is the attempt by one person to keep bad news from another, has been considered in terms of its function as an act of love or as the need to deny. Attempts to break collusion have been seen as a three-part process in which the aim is to promote mutual disclosure between a couple or a family.

The first stage is the need to assess the colluder and to attempt to identify the reasons for the collusion. In acknowledging the colluder's knowledge of the protected individual and by promising not to spell out bad news in a brutal way, it should be possible to negotiate access to the protected individual to assess their current knowledge of the situation and what they believe to be the current situation.

By talking to the protected person it is very common to find that they are aware of the bad news – for example, a diagnosis of cancer – but they too have not been talking to their loved one because they need to protect them from distressing information.

A third stage in the attempt to break collusion has been described, which is to get the couple together so that they can talk and discuss the current situation. The health professional may be able to withdraw once the subject has been brought up and the couple start to speak to each other, but experience has shown that if the first two stages are followed without an attempt to get the couple together, the collusion may remain intact and make it difficult for the couple to talk to each other and to deal with unfinished business.

It has been seen that if a couple are differential copers,

other methods may be required to meet the needs of each partner, and that collusion may continue in some situations.

HOPE

The need to consider hope within the framework of reality has been established. This moves hope from the narrow definition of hope for a total recovery from the bad news situation to hope within the constraints of the bad news. This allows for realistic reassurances to be given and short-term goals to be set.

It has been seen that in many bad news situations, the boundaries of hope may continue to move and possibly to contract as the level of bad news changes. An example of this is the dying patient who may not accept the bad news about their impending death and may be hoping to have a holiday. As adaptation to reality occurs, the hope may change to an outing with the family for a short period of time or the boundaries may be moved to such an extent that the hope is for an anniversary to be reached rather than anything more elaborate.

For that small percentage of people who cannot maintain hope and see their current situation as hopeless, the health professional needs to be alert to the possibility of clinical depression and suicidal thoughts.

UNFINISHED BUSINESS

Most individuals have things that are unsaid between themselves and those they love. A bad news situation can highlight unfinished business between individuals within a family and friendship circle. One thread throughout this book has emphasized helping the individual who receives bad news to adapt to that reality, for only then can unfinished business be approached.

Even when reality is faced, family members may find it difficult to talk to each other and to say the things that they have in the past been aware of but not made explicit. The importance of encouraging family members to talk to each other and to deal with unfinished business is bound up with the cost of missed opportunities. The 'if only' syndrome has been described, where individuals, particularly after a death, bemoan their lost opportunity to tell the dead person how much they were loved and how much they would be missed.

It can be very satisfying for a dying person to feel that they are in control of what is happening and that they can settle their business and know that their wishes will be observed. This is only possible with cooperation from loved ones.

The tasks of grieving have been described along with the concept that, after adaptation to bad news and the consequent feelings of grief, those who are adapting to bad news can move towards a more positive future.

THE MESSENGER

The emphasis on the messenger has dealt with the cost of bearing bad news and the need to know that any emotional reactions that are projected on to the messenger are not meant personally. To accept this, the messenger needs to have some insight and self-awareness of their own limits and strengths and vulnerabilities.

By learning to help individuals to focus their displaced emotions in a more appropriate place, the messenger can better handle the cost of giving bad news. Self-awareness may lead the messenger to develop an assertive approach when handling the difficulties with those who are reacting to bad news and feel the need to 'shoot the messenger.'

Survival strategies have been considered which help the professional to continue their work in a constructive way without the risk of burnout.

Index

Page references in **bold** indicate figures